Department of Health

362.14 DEP

Domiciliary Care

CHEADLE Library

National Minimum Standards

Regulations

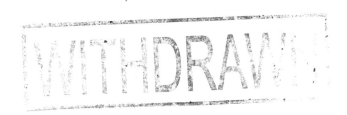

WITHDRAWN

London: TSO

Published by TSO (The Stationery Office) and available from:

Online
www.tso.co.uk/bookshop

Mail, Telephone, Fax & E-mail
TSO
PO Box 29, Norwich, NR3 1GN
Telephone orders/General enquiries: 0870 600 5522
Fax orders: 0870 600 5533
E-mail: book.orders@tso.co.uk
Textphone 0870 240 3701

TSO Shops
123 Kingsway, London, WC2B 6PQ
020 7242 6393 Fax 020 7242 6394
68-69 Bull Street, Birmingham B4 6AD
0121 236 9696 Fax 0121 236 9699
9-21 Princess Street, Manchester M60 8AS
0161 834 7201 Fax 0161 833 0634
16 Arthur Street, Belfast BT1 4GD
028 9023 8451 Fax 028 9023 5401
18-19 High Street, Cardiff CF10 1PT
029 2039 5548 Fax 029 2038 4347
71 Lothian Road, Edinburgh EH3 9AZ
0870 606 5566 Fax 0870 606 5588

TSO Accredited Agents
(see Yellow Pages)

and through good booksellers

Published with the permission of the Department of Health
on behalf of the Controller of Her Majesty's Stationery Office

First published 2003
Third impression 2005

ISBN 0 11 322545 8

Web Access
This document is available on the DoH internet website at:
http:/www.doh.gov.uk/ncsc

Printed in the United Kingdom for The Stationery Office
176164   C10   2/05

Contents

Appendices   **40**

National Minimum Standards for...   **50**

Statutory Instruments   **55**

Introduction

This document sets out the National Minimum Standards for domiciliary care agencies including local authority provision and NHS Trusts. They form the criteria by which the National Care Standards Commission will determine whether the agency provides personal care to the required standard. The purpose of these minimum standards is to ensure the quality of personal care and support which people receive whilst living in their own home in the community.

These standards establish the minimum required; ie they identify a standard of service provision below which an agency providing personal care for people living in their own home must not fall.

While broad in scope, these standards acknowledge the unique and complex needs of individuals, and the additional specific knowledge, and skills required in order to deliver a service that is tailored to the needs of each person. These standards will be applied to agencies providing personal care to the wide range of people who need care and support whilst living in their own home, including:

- older people

- people with physical disabilities

- people with sensory loss including dual sensory impairment

- people with mental health problems

- people with learning disabilities

- children and their families

- personal or family carers

Care and support workers may be directly providing the care themselves but they are more likely to be providing the care jointly with the person needing assistance, encouraging them to do as much as possible for themselves in order to maintain their independence and physical ability. Support workers will be providing support and assistance to people with a range of disabilities, helping them to maximise their own potential and independence. It is important that agencies and care workers who are providing personal domiciliary care for children and their families take note of the content of *Working Together to Safeguard Children* - a guide to inter-agency working to safeguard and promote the welfare of children.

With the emphasis on caring for people with complex health and personal care needs living in their own home instead of in residential or nursing homes or long stay hospitals, the provision of personal domiciliary care services is evolving rapidly and reflects changes at the interface between health and social care.

The Regulatory Context

These standards are published by the Secretary of State for Health in accordance with section 23 of the Care Standards Act 2000 (CSA) .

The CSA reforms the regulatory system for care services in England and Wales. It creates the National Care Standards Commission (NCSC), an independent, non-governmental public body, to regulate social and health care services previously regulated by local councils and health authorities. In addition, it extends the scope of regulation significantly to other services not currently registered, to include domiciliary care agencies, fostering agencies and residential family centres.

The CSA sets out abroad range of regulation making powers covering, amongst other matters, the management, staff, premises and conduct of social and healthcare establishments and agencies. Section 23 gives powers to the Secretary of State to publish statements of National Minimum Standards that the NCSC must take into account when making its decisions. These standards will form the basis for judgements made by the NCSC regarding registration and the imposition of conditions for registration, variation to any conditions and enforcement of compliance with the Care Standards Act 2000 and associated regulations, including proceedings for cancellation or prosecution.

The Commission will therefore consider the degree to which a regulated service complies with the standards when determining whether or not a service should be registered or have its registration cancelled, or whether to take any action for breach of regulations.

Who will be regulated?

Regulation applies to all agencies which provide personal care for persons living in their own homes who by reason of illness, infirmity or disability are unable to provide it for themselves without assistance. Agencies providing personal care at any time will need to register.

The term 'agency' includes all providers of personal domiciliary care services in the private, voluntary and public sectors including the local authority's own services, and NHS Trusts and supported housing or living schemes where applicable.

Definitions

Section 4(3) of the Care Standards Act defines domiciliary care agencies for the purposes of regulation by the Commission.

The following standards will NOT apply to employment agencies who solely act as introducers of workers employed by the user.

> **Standards 4, 5.2 only, 5.3 only, 6.3 only, 6.4 only, 7, 10.8 only, 10.9 only, 11, 12, 13, 14, 15, 16, 18, 19, 20, 21 and 24.1 bullet points 2, 5 and 9 only, 24.3, 24.4 and 27.3 bullet points 1 and 2 only. They are further exempt from bullet points 6, 11 and 13 onlyof Appendix B and all of Appendix F.**

The CSA sets out a broad range of regulation making powers covering, amongst other matters, the management, staff, premises and conduct of social and independent healthcare establishments and agencies. Section 23 gives powers to the Secretary of State to publish statements of national minimum standards that the NCSC must take into account when making its decisions. The standards will form the basis for judgements made by the NCSC regarding registration and the imposition of conditions for registration, variation of any conditions and enforcement of compliance with the CSA and associated Regulations, including proceedings for cancellation of registration or prosecution. The NCSC will therefore consider the degree to which a regulated service complies with the standards when determining whether or not a service should be registered or have its registration cancelled, or whether to take any action for breach of Regulations.

Where an agency operates from more than one branch, each branch will have to register and be inspected, and will also be required to have a responsible and registered 'fit manager' in charge of the day to day provision.

Where a national voluntary organisation has a number of affiliated branches, each of which is separately registered with the Charity Commission, each will be treated as a separate agency for the purposes of registration and regulation.

Where the business is a franchise operation, each individual franchise will be treated as a separate business.

The registered person and registered manager(s)

All agencies providing personal domiciliary care services, irrespective of size will be required to have a person as registered as the 'Fit Person' who has overall responsibility for the service.
This person may be the owner or the most senior manager of the service.

Where the Registered Person is not responsible for the day to day management of the service or where they lack the required qualifications and experience or where the service is provided from more than one office location, the Registered Person must appoint an experienced and qualified manager responsible for managing the office location on a day to day basis. This manager must also apply to be registered by the NCSC.

Definition of personal care

The Care Standards Act, 2000 did not include a definition of "personal care" (except that regulations may be made excluding prescribed activities from personal care). Its established, ordinary meaning includes four main types of care which are:

- assistance with bodily functions such as feeding, bathing and toileting

- care falling just short of assistance with bodily functions, but still involving physical and intimate touching, including activities such as helping a person get out of a bath and helping them to get dressed

- non-physical care, such as advice, encouragement and supervision relating to the foregoing, such as prompting a person to take a bath and supervising them during this

emotional and psychological support, including the promotion of social functioning, behaviour management, and assistance with cognitive functions.

NB: It is the Department's view, as reflected in the Guidance it has issued, that only the types of personal care set out in the first two bullet points above will give rise to registration as a domiciliary care agency under the Care Standards Act 2000. However, it is, of course, up to the National Care Standards Commission to decide (taking into account the facts of a particular case and the law} whether or not an undertaking is registrable as a domiciliary care agency, and if in doubt you should refer to them. In addition, the courts are likely to continue to define the term "personal care" as time goes by. Please refer to the Guidance - Supported Housing and Care Homes- Guidance on Regulation, httpll: www.doh.gov.uk/scg/shchguidance.htm where necessary.

Development of the standards

Stage one: The starting point was the analysis of existing voluntary regulatory and approved provider schemes. The common themes were extracted from over 90 schemes and examples of good practice identified in relation to each of the themes.

Stage two: An expert core working group of 20 people was assembled representing provider organisations from all sectors and including inspection and regulation and health service interest. The initial draft standards were developed and refined from the work of this group.

Stage three: The draft standards were then shared and discussed with representatives of service users and by a broad reference group of some 50 people and organisations. The standards were further refined as a result of the consultation and redrafted into a common format required for all the regulatory standards.

Stage four: The draft standards were published for consultation and revised to reflect the response prior to final publication.

Structure

The standards are grouped under five key topics and the outcome for service users identified in relation to each theme.

The topics are:

*   User focused services (Standards 1 - 6)

*   Personal care (Standards 7- 10)

*   Protection (Standards 11 - 16)

*   Managers and staff (Standards 17- 21)

*   Organisation and running of the business (Standards 22 - 27)

The standards have been designed to achieve the outcomes and to be enforceable through the relevant regulations. While the standards are qualitative - they provide a tool for judging the quality of care and support provided for service users - they are also measurable. Regulators will look for evidence that the requirements are being met and a good quality of life enjoyed by service users through:

- discussions with service users, families and friends, care and support staff, managers, and others

- observation of daily life in the home of the person receiving care and in the office of the organisation providing the service

- scrutiny of written policies, procedures, and records

The involvement of lay assessors in inspections will help ensure a focus on outcomes for and quality of life of service users.

The following cross-cutting themes underpin the drafting of the National Minimum Standards for the provision of personal domiciliary care services:

- **Focus on service users.** Modernising Social Services (1998) called for standards that "focus on the key areas that most affect the quality of life experienced by service users," [4.48] . The consultation process for developing the standards, and recent research, confirm the importance of this emphasis on results for service users. In applying the standards, regulators will look for evidence that the personal care and support is provided in such away that it achieves positive outcomes for and the active participation of service users.

- **Fitness for purpose.** The regulatory powers provided by the Care Standards Act are designed to ensure that organisations providing personal domiciliary care and the managers and care staff it employs are "fit for their purpose". In applying the standards, regulators will look for evidence that the organisation is successful in achieving its stated aims and objectives.

- **Comprehensiveness.** The provision of domiciliary care to anyone service user is made up of a range of separate but often related activities and services which will vary from person to person according to their needs. In applying the standards, regulators will consider how the total care package provided contributes to the overall personal and health care needs and preferences of service users, and how the organisation collaborates with other services / professionals to maximise independence and ensure the individual's inclusion in the community.

- **Meeting assessed needs.** In applying the standards, inspectors will look for evidence that the care provided meets the assessed needs of service users and that individuals' changing needs continue to be met. There should be a reassessment of need on an annual basis or more frequently if necessary. Inspectors will also wish to see evidence that care and support staff are able to be flexible to meet the changing needs and requirements of service users on a short term or temporary basis.

- **Quality services.** The Government's modernising agenda, including the new regulatory framework, aims to ensure "greater assurance of quality services. . .rather than having to live with second best". In applying the standards, regulators will seek evidence of a commitment to continuous improvement, quality services and support, which assure a good quality of life and health for service users and which contributes to maintaining their independence.

- **Quality workforce.** Competent, well-trained managers and staff are fundamental to achieving good quality care for service users. The Training Organisation for Personal Social Services, is developing National Occupational Standards for care and support staff, including induction competencies and foundation programmes. In applying the standards, regulators will look for evidence that registered managers and staff achieve the NTO requirements.

Context and purpose

These standards, and the regulatory framework within which they operate, should be viewed in the context of the Government's overall policy objectives for supporting people in their own home. These objectives emphasise the need to maintain and promote independence wherever possible, through rehabilitation and community support. A variety of specialist provision will be required to help achieve these objectives. The provision of high quality personal care to people living in their own homes will be the foundation of much of the specialist provision.

These standards have been prepared in response to extensive consultation and are realistic, proportionate, fair and transparent. They provide National Minimum Standards below which no provider may operate, ensure the protection of service users and safeguard and promote the health, welfare and quality of life of people living in their own home.

User focused services

Introduction to standards 1 – 6 (see user focused services section of the bibliography)

The needs of the service user lie at the heart of the provision of personal care. Service users need to be kept informed and enabled to make choices concerning their care, and participate in the process, thereby maintaining their independence. The service should be managed and provided at all times in a way which, meets the individual needs of the person receiving care, as specified in their care plan, and respects the rights, privacy and dignity of the individual.

Where the provision of personal domiciliary care is commissioned by the local authority, a three way working relationship should be developed with the local authority and the agency providing personal care working in partnership to most effectively meet the needs of the person requiring care.

In order to ensure that service users and/or their relatives or representatives are able to make informed choices concerning their care, they should be provided with a range of information that is up to date and is available in an appropriate language or format. A number of documents are required. Each has its own particular purpose.

Each agency providing personal domiciliary care should produce a guide for service users with a statement of purpose, setting out its aims and objectives, the range of services it offers and outlining the terms and conditions on which it does so. In this way service users, their relatives and representatives can make a fully informed choice about whether or not the organisation is suitable and able to meet the individual's particular needs. A copy of the most recent inspection report should also be made available. The statement of purpose will enable inspectors to assess how far the organisation's claims are being fulfiled.

Providing user focused services also means ensuring that care workers have the flexibility to vary the care provided to meet changing needs on a day to day basis. For example if the need is to assist the service user get up, washed and dressed and give them breakfast, the care worker must be able to respond flexibly and appropriately if on one occasion they find that they feel unwell and want to remain in bed.

Research into the views of service users about their personal care has identified that the continuity of care and support worker is extremely important. Service users and their relatives need to feel comfortable, relaxed and secure with the care workers they are inviting into their home. They want to have care workers they can get to know and who are reliable, dependable and arrive and depart at the time expected. Service users and their relatives also want to know in advance if there is to be any change in their care or support worker so they can be prepared.

Information

OUTCOME: Current and potential service users and their relatives have access to comprehensive information, so that they can make informed decisions on whether the agency is able to meet their specific care needs.

STANDARD 1 (See regulations 4 and 5)

1.1 **The registered person produces a Statement of Purpose and a Service User's Guide for current and prospective service users and their relatives. The contents of the Statement of Purpose are listed in Schedule I of the Regulations. The contents of the Service User's Guide must include those items listed in regulation 5. The Service User's Guide contains up to date information on the organisation setting out the aims, objectives, philosophy of care and parameters of the service provided, including terms and conditions. Also, the certificate of registration is prominently displayed at all times so as to be readily and easily seen in accordance with the Section 28(I) of the Care Standards Act.**

1.2 The Statement of Purpose and the Service User's Guide are written in plain English and are available in appropriate formats eg large print, braille. Where services are or may be provided to people for whom English is not their first language, the documents are made available in the language of their choice. The Service User's Guide includes:

- the aims and objectives of the agency

- the nature of the services provided, including specialist services

- people for whom the service is provided

- an overview of the process for the delivery of care and support from initial referral, through needs and risk assessment and development of the service user plan to review of the care and reassessment of need

- key contract terms and conditions

- the complaints procedure

- the Quality Assurance process

- specific information on key policies and procedures

- how to contact the local office of the National Care Standards Commission (NCSC), social services, health care authorities and the General Social Services Council (GSCC).

- hours of operation

- details of insurance cover

1.3 The registered person ensures that the Service User's Guide and the Statement of Purpose is dated, reviewed annually and updated as necessary.

1.4   All service users, their carers and prospective service users must be provided with the Service User's Guide and are informed that they may inspect the Agency's Statement of Purpose and how to access this document.

Care needs assessment

OUTCOME: The care needs requirements of service users and their personal or family carers when appropriate, are individually assessed before they are offered a personal domiciliary care service

STANDARD 2 (see regulation 14)

2.1   **A domiciliary care needs assessment regarding new service users is undertaken, prior to the provision of a domiciliary care service (or within 2 working days in exceptional circumstances), by people who are trained to do so, using appropriate methods of communication so that the service user and their representatives, are fully involved.**

2.2   The registered manager ensures that a care needs assessment is undertaken and obtains a summary of the needs assessment. For each user an assessment is obtained from either the local authority, health or primary care trust.

2.3   For individuals who are self-funding a care needs assessment is undertaken (appropriate to the level of support requested) in the individual's own home, by a manager competent and trained for the task, covering the delivery of the services agreed. Issues that may arise include:

- personal care and physical well-being

- family involvement and other personal and social contacts

- sight, hearing and communication

- continence

- mobility, dexterity and the need for disability equipment

- mental health and cognition

- medication requirements

- personal safety and risk

- specific condition-related needs and specialist input

- dietary requirements and preferences (if appropriate)

- social interests, religious and cultural needs (if appropriate)

- preferred method of communication

- method of payment

2.4 Information from the care needs assessment is provided in writing to care and support workers so that they are aware of any special needs, the activities they are required to undertake and the outcomes to be achieved.

2.5 When a service is provided at short notice or in a crisis, and a care needs assessment has not been undertaken, the person providing the service is trained and able to undertake an initial contact assessment if required.

2.6 Procedures are in place to enable care and support staff to report changes to the care needs and circumstances of service users and their carers so that a reassessment of care needs can be undertaken if necessary.

Meeting needs

> OUTCOME: Service users, their relatives and representatives know that the agency providing the personal care service has the skills and competence required to meet their care needs

STANDARD 3 (see regulation 14)

3.1 The registered person is able to demonstrate the capacity of the agency to meet the needs (including specialist needs) of individuals accepted by the agency.

3.2 Staff individually and collectively have the skills and experience to deliver the services and care which the agency states in its information material that it can provide. The skills and experience of care staff are matched to the care needs of each service user and they are able to communicate effectively with the service user using the individual's preferred method of communication.

3.3 All specialised services offered (and identified in the Service User's Guide) are demonstrably based on current good practice, relevant to the agency, and reflect relevant specialist and clinical guidance. This includes specialist services for people with dementia, mental health problems, sensory impairment, physical disabilities, learning disabilities, substance misuse problems, intermediate or respite care.

3.4 When services are provided for specific minority ethnic communities, social/cultural or religious groups their particular requirements and preferences are identified, understood and entered into a plan for the servIce user.

Contract

> OUTCOME: Each service user has a written individual service contract or equivalent for the provision of care, with the agency, except employment agencies solely introducing workers.

STANDARD 4

4.1 **Each service user is issued with a written contract (if self -funding) provided by the agency within seven days of commencement of the service.**

4.2   The contract between the service user and the service provider specifies the following, unless these appear in the Service User's Guide and Care Plan:

- name, address and telephone number of agency

- contact number for out of hours and details of how to access the service.

- contact number for the office of regular care workers and their manager

- areas of activity which home care or support workers will and will not undertake and the degree of flexibility in the provision of personal care.

- circumstances in which the service may be cancelled or withdrawn including temporary cancellation by the service user

- fees payable for the service, and by whom

- rights and responsibilities of both parties (including insurance) and liability if there is a breach of contract or any damage occurring in the home

- arrangements for monitoring and review of needs and for updating the assessment (see Standard 2) and the individual service user plan (see Standard 7)

- process for assuring the quality of the service, monitoring and supervision of staff

- supplies and/or equipment to be made available by the service user and by the agency

- respective responsibilities of the service user and of the agency in rel:ltion to health and safety matters

- arrangements to cover holidays and sickness

- keyholding and other arrangements agreed for entering or leaving the home (see Standard 15)

4.3   The service user and/or their relatives or representative and the agency each has a copy of the contract which is signed by the service user (or their named representative on their behalf) and the registered manager.

Confidentiality (see regulation 13)

OUTCOME: Service users and their relatives or representatives know that their personal information is handled appropriately and that their personal confidences are respected. In the case of standards 5.2 and 5.3, these do not apply to employment agencies solely introducing workers.

STANDARD 5

5.1   **Care and support staff respect information given by service users or their representatives in confidence and handle information about service users in accordance with the Data Protection Act 1998 and the agency's written policies and procedures and in the best interests of the service user.**

5.2   Service users have summaries of the agency's policies and procedures on confidentiality which specifies the circumstances under which confidentiality may be breached and includes the process for dealing with inappropriate breaches of confidentiality.

5.3   Care or support workers know when information given them in confidence must be shared with their manager and other social/health care agencies.

5.4   The principles of confidentiality are observed in discussion with colleagues and the line manager, particularly when undertaking training or group supervision sessions.

5.5   Suitable provision is made for the safe and confidential storage of service user records and information including the provision of lockable filing cabinets and the shielding of computer screens from general view when displaying personal data.

Responsive services

OUTCOME: Service users receive a flexible, consistent and reliable personal care service. In the case of standards 6.3 and 6.4 these do not apply to employment agencies solely introducing workers.

STANDARD 6 (see standard 15)

6.1   Staff are reliable and dependable, are able to respond flexibly to the needs and preferences of service users which arise on a day to day basis and services are provided in a way that meets the outcomes identified in the care plan.

6.2   Staff arrive at the home within the time band specified and work for the full amount of time allocated.

6.3   Upon arrival in the home, care or support staff ask the service user if there are any particular personal care needs or requirements they have on that visit.

6.4   The registered manager ensures that there is continuity in relation to the care or support worker(s) who provide(s) the service to each service user.

6.5   Care or support workers are only changed for legitimate reasons for example:

   •   the care or support worker is sick, on holiday, undertaking training or has left the organisation

   •   if the service requirements change and the care worker does not have the necessary skills, physical capacity or specialist training

   •   the care or support worker is unavailable for additional hours or changed times

   •   if the service user requests a change of care or support worker for legitimate reasons

   •   if a non-professional relationship has developed between the service user and the care or support worker.

   •   to provide relief for care or support staff working in stressful situations

- to protect care or support staff from abuse, discrimination

6.6   Service users their relatives or representatives are consulted in advance whenever possible, and involved in the decision about the change of care or support worker, if the change is permanent or likely to last longer than 30 days.

6.7   Service users, their relatives and/or representatives are kept fully informed on issues relating to their care, at all times.

Personal care

Introduction to standards 7 – 10 (see personal care section of bibliography)

The principles on which the philosophy of care of the provider organisation is based must be ones which ensure that all service users, their relatives and representatives are treated with respect, their dignity is preserved at all times and their right to privacy is always observed. The test of whether these principles are put into practice or not will be a matter for each person's own judgement: Care and support workers should put themselves in the place of people receiving care and ask themselves:

- how am I treated by home care staff when they are bathing me and helping me dress?

- how do they speak to me?

- am I consulted in matters to do with my own care and am I able to make choices?

- are my wishes respected?

- are my views taken into account?

Fundamentally care and support workers should 'treat others as you would wish to be treated yourself'.

The purpose of the provision of personal care to people who are living in their own home is to sustain and whenever possible improve their independence. As well as ensuring their involvement in all decisions relating to their care this also means involving them and supporting them to assist in the care activities themselves rather than increasing dependence by taking over and doing everything for them.

The provision of personal care for people who live in their own homes is changing. The interface between health and personal care is becoming very blurred. Meeting the Government agenda on intermediate care, maintaining independence and partnership working will further contribute to a confusion of role between health care professionals and personal social care. As the health and care needs of people living in their own home become more complex, so home care and support staff come under pressure to undertake increasingly complex health related activities. This should never happen 'by default' but only with the written agreement of all parties and when the home care or support worker has received the appropriate and necessary training. Clarity in the roles, if any, in relation to medication and other health related activities is therefore essential.

Service user plan

OUTCOME: The care needs, wishes, preferences and personal goals for each individual service user are recorded in their personal service user plan, except for employment agencies solely introducing workers.

STANDARD 7 (See regulation 14)

7.1 **A personal service user plan outlining the delivery arrangements for the care is developed and agreed with each service user, which provides the basis for the care to be delivered and is generated from the care needs assessment, (Standard 2) service user plan, risk and manual handling risk assessment (Standard 12) and the service contract or statement of terms and conditions. (Standard 4)**

7.2 The plan sets out in detail the action that will be taken by care and support workers to meet the assessed needs, including specialist needs and communication requirements, and identifies areas of flexibility to enable the service user maximise their potential and maintain their independence. (see Standards 6 & 9)

7.3 The plan is drawn up with the involvement of the service user, whenever possible or their representative on their behalf, their relatives and friends and any other professional as appropriate and takes into account the service user's wishes and preferences in relation to the way in which the care is provided and their own chosen lifestyle - as long as it conforms to legal requirements and does not compromise the provider agencys' obligations.

7.4 The plan establishes individualised procedures for service users in relation to the taking of risks in daily living and for those service users who are likely to be aggressive, abusive or cause harm or self-harm, focussing on positive behaviour. (See Standards 9.8,12 and 14.6)

7.5 The information and detail provided in the plan is appropriate for the complexity of the service to be provided.

7.6 The plan is reviewed as changes in circumstances require but at least annually with the service user, their relatives, friends and significant professionals or at the request of the service user or their representative or if there has been a change in their care needs and/or circumstances of the service user or their carer. The plan is updated and agreed changes are recorded and actioned.

7.7 The plan is signed by the service user or their representative on their behalf and is available in a language and format that the service user can understand. A copy of the plan is held by the service user unless there are clear and recorded reasons not to do so.

Private and Dignity

OUTCOME: Service users feel that they are treated with respect and valued as a person, and their right to privacy is upheld

STANDARD 8 (See regulation 14)

8.1 **Personal care and support is provided in a way which maintains and respects the privacy, dignity and lifestyle of the person receiving care at all times with particular regard to assisting with:**

- **dressing and undressing**

- **bathing, washing, shaving and oral hygiene**

- **toilet and continence requirements**

- **medication requirements and other health related activities**

- **manual handling**

- **eating and meals**

- **handling personal possessions and documents**

- **entering the home, room, bathroom or toilet**

8.2 Care and support is provided in the least intrusive way at all times.

8.3 Service users, their relatives and their representative are treated with courtesy at all times.

8.4 Service users are addressed by the name they prefer at all times.

8.5 Care and support workers are sensitive and responsive to the race, culture, religion, age, disability, gender and sexuality of the people receiving care, and their relatives and representatives.

Autonomy and independence

OUTCOME: Service users are assisted to make their own decisions and control their own lives and are supported in maintaining their independence

STANDARD 9 (See regulation 14)

9.1 **Managers and care and support workers enable service users to make decisions in relation to their own lives, providing information, assistance, and support where needed.**

9.2 Service users are encouraged, enabled and empowered to control their personal finances unless prevented from doing so by severe mental incapacity or disability. (see Standard 13.5)

9.3   Care and support workers carry out tasks *with* the service user, not *for* them, minimising the intervention and supporting service users to take risks, as set out in the service user plan, and not endangering health and safety. (see Standards 7 & 12)

9.4   When caring for children, opportunity is taken to enable them to participate in the activity and to develop through learning and playing, and to protect them from abuse or harm.

9.5   Service users, and their relatives and representatives are kept fully informed about the service they receive and are provided with information in an appropriate format.

9.6   Care and support workers communicate with service users in the their first or, where agreed, their preferred language.

9.7   Service users or their relatives or representatives (with permission of the service user) are able to see their personal files kept on the premises of the provider agency, in accordance with the Data Protection Act 1998 and are informed in writing that these files may be reviewed as part of the inspection and regulation process. (see Standard 24)

9.8   Limitations on the chosen lifestyle or human rights to prevent self-harm or self-neglect, or abuse or harm to others, are made only in the service user's best interest, consistent with the agency's responsibilities in law. The limitations are recorded in full within the risk assessment and the plan for managing the risks (see Standard 1 2) and entered into the service user plan. (see Standard 7)

9.9   Service users and their relatives or other representatives are informed about independent advocates who will act on their behalf and about self-advocacy schemes.

Medication and health related activities

OUTCOME: The agency's policy and procedures on medication and health related activities protect service users and assists them to maintain responsibility for their own medication and to remain in their own home, even if they are unable to administer their medication themselves. In the case of standards 10.8, and 10.9, these do not apply to employment agencies solely introducing workers.

STANDARD 10 (See regulation 14)

10.1   **The registered person ensures there is a clear, written policy and procedure which is adhered to by staff and which identifies parameters and circumstances for assisting with medication and health related tasks and identifies the limits to assistance and tasks which may not be undertaken without specialist training.**

10.2   The policy should include procedures if required for obtaining prescriptions and dispensed medicines and for recording the information.

10.3   Staff only provide assistance with taking medication or administer medication or undertake other health related tasks, when it is within their competence; they have received any necessary specialist training and it is:

•   **with the informed consent of the service user or their relatives or representative**

- clearly requested on the care plan by a named assessor

- with agreement of the care or support workers' line manager, and

- not contrary to the agency's policy

10.4   Assistance with medication and other health related activities is identified in the Care Plan, forms part of the risk assessment (Standard 12) and is detailed within the Service User Plan.

10.5   Care and support staff leave medication at all times in a safe place which is known and accessible to the service user or, if not appropriate for the service user to have access, where it is only accessible to relatives and other personal carers, health personnel and domiciliary care staff.

10.6   Care and support workers follow the agency's procedures for reporting concerns, responding to incidents and seeking guidance.

10.7   Care and support workers record, with the user's permission, observation of the service user taking medication and any assistance given, including dosage and time of medication and undertaking any other health related tasks, on the record of the care visit kept in the home and/or the Home Care Medication record and the personal file of the service user held in the agency. Any advice to the service user to see or call in their General Practitioner or other health care professional is also recorded. The record is signed and dated by the care worker and the service user or their representative.

10.8   Except for employment agencies solely introducing workers, where delivery of the care package involves multiple agencies, including health care, a policy on medication and health related tasks is agreed and followed. A key worker, generally a health care professional from one agency who visits on a regular basis is identified as responsible for taking the lead on medication. Care and support workers retain responsibility for their own actions in accordance with the policy.

10.9   Except for employment agencies solely introducing workers, where necessary and agreed the policy and procedures are approved by a suitably experienced pharmacist, if appropriate. The functions undertaken by staff in this context need to be covered by the employers insurance policy.

Protection

Introduction to Standards 11 – 15 (See protective section bibliography)

Health and Safety

The health and safety of service users and home care and support workers is a major issue of concern in the provision of personal domiciliary care. Despite the requirements of legislation, accidents occur all too frequently. Failure to observe health and safety requirements is a major cause of long term illness among home care staff. Training on all aspects of health and safety is essential to ensure that home care and support staff are able to respond appropriately and work in a safe manner.

Before commencing the provision of care in a new home, to comply with the requirements of legislation a detailed risk assessment must be made by the organisation providing the service, of the risks associated with the delivery of the service. This assessment must be undertaken by someone who is trained for the purpose. This may be the registered manager or it may be an experienced home care or support worker. The risk assessment must be comprehensive and include, where appropriate, the risks associated with assisting with medication as well as any risks associated with travelling to and from the home of the service user, particularly late at night.

A separate assessment must be undertaken of the risks associated with manual handling. It is important that care strategies are devised in relation to assisting people with disabilities which are acceptable to the person concerned and are also safe for the care and support workers involved. Guidance on manual handling from the Health and Safety Executive has been revised and updated in 2002. The Department of Health guidance on Fair Access to Care Services was published in 2002.

The service user also retains responsibilities in relation to the health and safety of the environment in which they live and not place people visiting the home at risk. All the risks identified must therefore be discussed in full with the service user, their relatives or representative, the home care or support worker and their line manager and the commissioner of the care (if involved). A plan to manage the identified risks must be compiled and agreed by all parties. The plan should include review and reassessment of the risks.

Protection of the person from abuse or exploitation

The general public is aware of the effects of child abuse; far less publicity is given to adult and elder abuse and many people, even those employed in providing care to adults, are still relatively unaware of the existence of abuse and its effects. Home care and support workers need to be aware that abuse does not have to be extreme or obvious. It can be unintentional, insidious and the cumulative result of ongoing bad practice. No organisation that is concerned with maintaining standards in the provision of professional care services can afford to ignore any form of abuse which affects the well being of the people for whom they are responsible.

The role that home care and support workers play in the lives of people they care for, is extremely important. It is the home care workers and support workers who have a key role in recognising and protecting people from abuse. They have a responsibility to the people for whom they provide the care service, to minimise both the likelihood of abusive situations occurring and the effects that it can have, and to contribute to monitoring anyone who may be considered to be 'at risk.'

It is essential that care is taken in all financial transactions undertaken on behalf of the service user and a full written record kept to safeguard both the service user and the home care or support worker and to ensure no misunderstandings occur. For similar reasons home care or support workers must never seek to profit from the care they provide to service users by the acceptance of significant gifts or bequests.

The safety of service users is very important and for this reason care must be taken when entering or leaving the premises of people receiving care. This includes the need to carry and show proper identification at all times.

Safe working practices

OUTCOME: The health, safety and welfare of service users and care and support staff is promoted and protected, except for employment agencies solely introducing workers.

STANDARD 11 (See regulations 12, 13, 14 and 15)

11.1   **The registered person ensures that the agency has systems and procedures in place to comply with the requirements of the Health and Safety legislation Including:**

- **Management of Health and Safety at Work Regulations 1999 (Management Regulations)**

- **Manual Handling Operations Regulations 1992**

- **Control of Substances Hazardous to Health Regulations (COSHH).**

- **Reporting of Injuries, Diseases and Dangerous Occurrences Regulations 1995 (RIDDOR)**

- **Lifting Operations and Lifting Equipment Regulations 1998 (LOLER)**

- **Provision and Use of Work Equipment Regulations 1998 (PUWER)**

- **Health and Safety at Work Act 1974**

- **Food Safety Act 1990**

11.2   The agency has a comprehensive health and safety policy, and written procedures for health and safety management defining:

- individual and organisational responsibilities for health & safety matters

- responsibilities and arrangements for risk assessment under the requirements of the Management of Health and Safety at Work Regulations 1999 (Management Regulations)

- arrangements to implement safe systems of work to safeguard the welfare of service users, staff and others involved in the provision of domiciliary care, taking into account the findings of the risk assessments

- procedures to be followed when safe systems of work identified as necessary to safeguard the service users, staff and others involved in the provision of domiciliary care, cannot be implemented

- responsibility and procedure for reporting and investigating accidents and dangerous occurrences including those specified under RIDDOR for both service users and staff

- reporting procedure to follow when either a service user or a member of staff has a known transmittable disease or infection

- the provision and wearing of protective clothing

- procedures for managing threats or violence to staff

- content of training on health and safety to be given to care and support workers (see Standard 19 and appendix D)

11.3   The registered person appoints one or more competent persons to assist the agency in complying with their health and safety duties and responsibilities including:

- identifying hazards and assessing risks

- preparing health and safety policy statements

- introducing risk control measures

- providing adequate training and refresher training

11.4   All organisational records relating to health and safety matters are accurate and kept up to date. (see Standard 24)

Risk assessment

OUTCOME: The risk of accidents and harm happening to Service Users and staff in the provision of the personal care, is minimised, except for employment agencies solely introducing workers.

STANDARD 12 (See regulation 14)

12.1   **The registered person ensures that an assessment is undertaken, by a trained and qualified person, of the potential risks to service users and staff associated with delivering the package of care, (including, where appropriate, the risks associated with assisting with medication and other health related activities} before the care or support worker commences work and is updated annually or more frequently if necessary.**

12.2   The risk assessment includes an assessment of the risks for service users in maintaining their independence and daily living within the home. (See Standard 7)

12.3   The manner in which the risk assessment is undertaken is appropriate to the needs of the individual service user and the views of the service user and their relatives are taken into account.

12.4   The registered person ensures that a separate moving and handling risk assessment is undertaken by a member of staff who is trained for the purpose, whenever staff are required to help a user with any manual handling task, as required under the Manual Handling Operations Regulations 1992.

12.5   A comprehensive plan to manage the risks including manual handling and the risks to service users, is drawn up in consultation with the service user, their relatives or representatives, included in the service user plan and kept in the home of the service user for staff to refer to. A copy is also placed on the personal file kept in the agency. The risk management plan is implemented and reviewed annually or more frequently if necessary.

12.6   A procedure is in place for reporting new risks which arise including defective appliances, equipment, fixtures or security of the premises.

12.7   Only staff who are both trained to undertake risk assessments and competent to provide the care are assigned to emergency situations and where pressure of time does not allow a risk assessment to be undertaken prior to provision of the care or support.

12.8   Two people fully trained in current safe handling techniques and the equipment to be used are always involved in the provision of care when the need is identified from the manual handling risk assessment.

12.9   The name and contact number of the organisation responsible for providing and maintaining any equipment under the Manual Handling Regulations and Lifting Operations and Lifting Equipment Regulations is recorded on the risk assessment.

12.10   The registered manager ensures that the manual handling equipment is in a safe condition to use, that inspections by the manufacturers have taken place on time and if necessary reminds the organisation providing the equipment that a maintenance check is due.

12.11   The registered person produces and ensures compliance with safety policies and procedures to protect staff travelling to and from the homes of service users including advice on eg:

•   not carrying large sums of money or medicines late at night

•   working in pairs

•   use of bleeps/pagers

•   use of mobile telephones

•   car insurance for business use

12.12   A responsible and competent person is on call and contactable at all times when care and support staff are on duty.

Financial protection

OUTCOME: The money and property of service users is protected at all times whilst providing the care service, except for employment agencies solely introducing workers.

STANDARD 13 (see regulation 14)

13.1 **The registered person ensures that there is a policy and there are procedures in place for staff on the safe handling of service users' money and property covering:**

- **payment for the service/ service user's contribution (if appropriate)**

- **payment of bills**

- **shopping**

- **collection of pensions**

- **safeguarding the property of service users whilst undertaking the care tasks**

- **reporting the loss or damage to property whilst providing the care**

and guidance on NOT:

- **accepting gifts or cash (beyond a very minimal value)**

- **using loyalty cards except those belonging to the service user**

- **making personal use of the service users property, eg telephone**

- **involving the service user in gambling syndicates (eg national lottery, football pools)**

- **borrowing or lending money**

- **selling or disposing of goods belonging to the service user and their family**

- **selling goods or services to the service user**

- **incurring a liability on behalf of the service user**

- **taking responsibility for looking after any valuable on behalf of the service user**

- **taking any unauthorised person (including children) or pets into the service user's home without permission of the service user, their relatives or representative and the manager of the service**

13.2 The agency's policies and practices regarding service users wills and bequests preclude the involvement of any staff or members of their family, in the making of or benefiting from service users wills or soliciting any other form of bequest or legacy or acting as witness or executor or being involved in any way with any other legal document.

13.3 The registered person ensures there is a policy and procedure for the investigation of allegations of financial irregularities and the involvement of police, social services and professional bodies.

13.4 The amount and purpose of all financial transactions undertaken on behalf of the service user, including shopping and the collection of pensions is recorded appropriately on the visit record held in the service users home (see Standard 16) and signed and dated by the care and support worker and by the service user, if able to do so, or their relatives or representatives on their behalf.

13.5 Where service users are unable to take responsibility for the management of their own finances, this is recorded on the risk assessment and action taken to minimise the risk. (See Standard 9.2)

13.6 The registered person will keep a register that is open to inspection and owners and managers will declare in writing in the register any interest or involvement with any other separate organisation providing care or support services or responsible for commissioning or contracting those services, including where partners or other close family members own or manage at a senior level, other businesses providing domiciliary, day, residential or nursing care.

Protection of the person

OUTCOME: Service users are protected from abuse, neglect and self-harm, except for employment agencies solely introducing workers.

STANDARD 14 (See regulation 14)

14.1 **Service users are safeguarded &om any form of abuse or exploitation including physical, financial, psychological, sexual abuse, neglect, discriminatory abuse or self-harm or inhuman or degrading treatment through deliberate intent, negligence or ignorance in accordance with written policies and procedures.**

14.2 The Registered Person ensures that the agency has robust procedures for responding to suspicion or evidence of abuse or neglect (including whistle blowing) to ensure the safety and protection of service users. The procedures reflect local multi-agency policies and procedures including the involvement of the Police and the passing on concerns to the NCSC in accordance with the Public Interest Disclosure Act 1998 and the Department of Health guidance No Secrets.

14.3 All allegations and incidents of abuse are followed up promptly and the details and action taken recorded in a special record/file kept for the purpose and on the personal file of the service user.

14.4 The Registered Person ensures that there is a detailed policy, and there are procedures and a management and reporting plan for child protection.

14.5 The Registered Manager ensures that care and support staff working with children and their families have copies of the local authority child protection procedures and are fully conversant with the agency's policy and procedures.

14.6 Physical and verbal aggression by a service user, their relatives or friends is responded to appropriately. Physical intervention is only used as a last resort, in accordance with Department of Health guidance and protects the rights and best interests of the service user, including people with special needs and is the minimum necessary consistent with safety. (see Standards 7.4 and 12)

14.7 Training on prevention of abuse is given to all staff within 6 months of employment and is updated every two years.

14.8 Staff who may be unsuitable to work with children are referred, in accordance with the Care Standards Act, for consideration for inclusion on the Protection of Children list.

Security of the home

OUTCOME: Service users are protected and are safe and secure in their home, except for employment agencies solely introducing workers.

STANDARD 15 (See regulation 14}

15.1 Care and support workers ensure the security and safety of the home and the service user at all times when providing personal care.

15.2 Clear protocols are in place in relation to entering the homes of service users which cover:

- knocking/ringing bell and speaking out before entry
- written and signed agreements on keyholding
- safe handling and storage of keys outside the home
- confidentiality of entry codes
- alternative arrangements for entering the home
- action to take in case of loss or theft of keys
- action to take when unable to gain entry
- securing doors and windows
- discovery of an accident to the service user
- other emergency situations

(See Standard 4.2)

15.3 Identity cards are provided for all care and support staff entering the home of service users. The cards should display:

- a photograph of the member of staff
- the name of the person and employing organisation in large print
- the contact number of the organisation

- date of issue and an expiry date which should not exceed 36 months from the date of issue

The cards should be:

- available in large print for people with visual disabilities

- laminated or otherwise tamper proof

- renewed and replaced within at least 36 months from the date of issue.

- returned to the organisation when employment ceases

15.4 For people with special communication requirements, there are clear and agreed ways of identifying care and support staff from the agency.

Records kept in the home

OUTCOME: The health, rights and best interests of service users are safeguarded by maintaining a record of key events and activities undertaken in the home in relation to the provision of personal care, except for employment agencies solely introducing workers.

STANDARD 16 (See regulation 18)

16.1 **With the users consent care or support workers record on records kept in the home of service users, the time and date of every visit of to the home, the service provided and any significant occurrence. Where employed by the agency, live-in care and support workers complete the record on a daily basis. Records include (where appropriate:**

- assistance with medication including time and dosage on a special medication chart. (See Standard 10)

- other requests for assistance with medication and action taken (See Standard 10)

- financial transactions undertaken on behalf of the service user (See Standard 13)

- details of any changes in the users or carers circumstances, health, physical condition and care needs

- any accident, however minor, to the service user and/or care or support worker

- any other untoward incidents

- any other information which would assist the next health or social care worker to ensure consistency in the provision of care

16.2 Service users and/or their relatives or representatives are informed about what is written on the record and have access to it.

16.3 All written records are legible, factual, signed and dated and kept in a safe place in the home, as agreed with the service user, their relatives or representative.

16.4 Records are kept in the home for one month, or until the service is concluded, after which time they are transferred, with the permission of the service user, to the provider agency or other suitable body (eg local authority or health trust, or other purchaser of the service), for safe keeping.

16.5 Any service user or their relatives or representative on their behalf, refusing to have records kept in their home, is requested to sign and date a statement confirming the refusal and this is kept on their personal file in the agency.

Managers and staff

Introduction to standards 17- 21 (See managers and staff section of bibliography)

The expectations that service users and their families have of home care and support staff is very high. The work places considerable responsibility on all home carers who work, predominantly on their own, in other peoples own homes and in unsupervised settings. The quality of the care provided to service users will directly reflect the calibre of staff employed and their level of competence. It is therefore essential that the people who are recruited to undertake the work are suitable for task. It is also essential that they are able to demonstrate their competence for the work they are employed to undertake. This means ensuring staff at all levels have opportunities to develop and receive the training necessary. 10 do otherwise would mean providing people living in their own home and requiring personal care with a second-rate' service.

As the care needs of people living at home become increasingly complex and as more people are discharged early from hospital, so there is a commensurate increase in the need for specialist training to meet the particular care needs of people with certain conditions. Training must also consider the needs of family and other carers.

The quality of care provided is strongly influenced by the calibre of the managers of the service. It is therefore important that they are also able to demonstrate their management competence and their ability to perform their responsibilities effectively. One of these responsibilities is the regular supervision and appraisal of staff This is particularly essential for home care staff who work daily in stressful, but totally unsupervised work settings. Unfortunately things do go wrong from time to time, and to deal with these situations it is necessary to have an effective disciplinary and grievance procedure. A Staff Handbook issued to all staff helps to ensure that they know what is expected of them and what they should do in certain critical situations. It is also important that it is realised that the application of the standards applies equally to the engagement of temporary or agency staff

Recruitment and selection

OUTCOME: The well-being, health and security of service users is protected by the agency's policies and procedures on recruitment and selection of staff

STANDARD 17 (See regulations 15 and 16)

17.1 **There is a rigorous recruitment and selection procedure which meets the requirements of legislation, equal opportunities and anti discriminatory practice and ensures the protection of service users and their relatives.**

17.2 Face to face selection interviews are undertaken on premises which are secure and private, for all staff (including volunteers) who are shortlisted and may be engaged.

17.3   Two written references are obtained before making an appointment, one of whom should normally be the immediate past employer and are followed up by a telephone call prior to confirmation of employment. Any gaps in the employment record are explored.

17.4   New staff and volunteers are confirmed in post only following completion of satisfactory checks. These checks include:

- verification of identity

- POCA list (where the post applied for is a "regulated position"

- work permit (if appropriate)

- driving licence (if appropriate)

- certificates of training and qualifications claimed

- declaration of physical and mental fitness

- confirmation service check by UKCC (if holding a nursing, midwifery or health visitor qualification)

- sex offenders register

- General Social Care Council Register

17.5   Checks on the suitability of temporary staff may be undertaken by an employment or recruitment agency on behalf of the provider agency, provided that the checks comply with the requirements of these standards.

17.6   New staff, including temporary workers and volunteers, are provided with a written contract specifying the terms and conditions under which they are engaged, including the need to comply with the agencies' Staff Handbook for staff. (See Standard 25)

17.7   Staff are employed in accordance with the code of conduct and practice set by the General Social Care Council and are given copies of the code.

17.8   The registered person complies with any Code of Practice published by the General Social Care Council setting out standards expected of persons employing social care workers, insofar as the code is relevant to the management of domiciliary care.

17.9   Staff are required to provide a statement that they have no criminal convictions, or to provide a statement of any criminal convictions that they do have.

Requirements of the job

OUTCOME: Service users benefit from clarity of staff roles and responsibilities, except for employment agencies solely introducing workers.

STANDARD 18 (See regulation 16)

18.1 **All managers and staff are provided with a written job description person and work specification, identifying their responsibilities and accountabilities and with copies of the organisations' Staff Handbook and grievance and disciplinary procedure.**

18.2 The person specification includes the personal qualities required to undertake the work and the appropriate attitudes to be adopted.

18.3 Activities which should not be undertaken by care and support staff are also identified.

18.4 Person and work specifications are developed with reference to the relevant National Occupational Standards.

18.5 Staff are required to notify their employer of any new criminal offence they may have committed, including motoring offences.

18.6 An immediate investigation is undertaken on any allegations or incidents of misconduct and appropriate disciplinary action taken as necessary.

18.7 A record is kept of all disciplinary incidents and details entered in the personal file of the member of staff concerned.

18.8 Staff who are believed to have committed any offence prescribed by regulations are immediately reported to the Protection of Children (POCA) list. (See Standard 14.8) , and, when it becomes operational, the Protection of Vulnerable Adults (POVA) list.

Development and training

OUTCOME: Service users know that staff are appropriately trained to meet their personal care needs, except for employment agencies solely introducing workers.

STANDARD 19 (See regulation 15)

19.1 **The registered person ensures that there is a staff development and training programme within the agency, reviewed and updated annually, which meets the workforce training targets of the Training Organisation for Personal Social Services, and ensures staff are able to fulfil the aims of the agency and meets the changing needs of service users, their relatives and representatives.**

19.2 There is a structured induction process, which is completed by new care and support staff, which encompasses the Training Organisation for Personal Social Services induction standards.

19.3 The induction process includes a minimum 3 days orientation programme at the start of employment which covers the topics to be found in appendix C and includes shadowing an experienced care or support worker prior to taking responsibility themselves for the provision of personal care services and working alone in the homes of service users.

19.4 Each new member of staff undertakes a training needs analysis on completion of induction or probationary period. This is incorporated into the staff training and development plan.

19.5 All staff are provided with the required training on health and safety including manual handling. Topics to be covered may be found in appendix D. (See Standard 11)

19.6 Specialist advice, training and information is provided for care or support workers working with specific user groups and/or medical conditions by someone who is professionally qualified to do so. A list of areas of specialist training need appears in appendix E.

19.7 Within the whole staff group there is the range of skills and competence required to work with and meet the needs of individual service users served by the agency. (See Standard 3)

19.8 Managers or supervisors of care or support workers providing specialist care services have knowledge and understanding of the specialisms for which they are responsible.

19.9 The agency has financial resources allocated, plans and operational procedures to achieve and monitor the requirements for workforce training and qualification.

19.10 The need for refresher and updating training is identified at least annually during staff appraisal (See Standard 21) and incorporated into the staff development and training programme.

Qualifications

OUTCOME: The personal care of service users is provided by qualified and competent staff, except for employment agencies solely introducing workers.

STANDARD 20 (See regulation 15)

20.1 **All staff in the organisation are competent and trained to undertake the activities for which they are employed and responsible.**

20.2 Newly appointed care or support workers delivering personal care who do not already hold a relevant care qualification are required to demonstrate their competence and register for the relevant NVQ in care award (either NVQ in Care level 2 or level 3) within the first six months of employment and complete the full award within three years. This standard will be deemed unmet if employers attempt simply to dismiss staff and re-hire every 6 months.

20.3 Unqualified staff employed for less than 2 years at the commencement of the application of the standards are phased into the relevant NVQ in care over the following 2 years and complete the award within 3 years.

20.4 50% of all personal care by the provider to be delivered by workers NVQ qualified or equivalent, or better, by Ist Apri12008. A detailed review of this target to be made available by Ist July 2006 so as to assess progress. Further reviews annually to set targets for 2 years hence. New personal care staff must continue to take up the NVQ course even when the 50% target has been reached.

20.5   Managers obtain a nationally recognised management qualification equivalent to NVQ level 4 in management within 5 years from the date of application of these standards, or following that period, within three years of employment.

20.6   Records of training and development undertaken and the outcome, are kept on a central development file and on individual personnel files.

20.7   Managers undertake periodic management training to update his or her knowledge, skills and competence to manage the agency.

Supervision

OUTCOME: Service users know and benefit from having staff who are supervised and whose performance is appraised regularly, except for employment agencies solely introducing workers.

STANDARD 21 (See regulation 15)

21.1   **All care and support staff receive regular supervision and have their standard of practice appraised annually.**

21.2   All staff meet formally on a one to one basis with their line manager to discuss their work at least 3 monthly and written records kept on the content and outcome of each meeting. (See Standard 27.3)

21.3   With the consent of the service user, at least one of these meetings should incorporate direct observation of the care worker providing care to a service user with whom they regularly work.

21.4   Regular meetings are also held at least quarterly with peers and/or other team members.

21.5   All staff have an annual appraisal of their overall standard of performance and identification of training and development needs, and a copy of the appraisal is placed on the personnel file of each care or support worker. The appraisal would normally be undertaken by the line manager or their manager, except in exceptional circumstances.

21.6   Managers and supervisors receive training in supervision skills and undertaking performance appraisal.

Organisation & running of the business

Introduction to standards 22-27 (see organisation section of bibliography)

It is essential that the organisations providing domiciliary care operate from a sound business basis in order to ensure that the provider organisation is able to meet the needs of service users efficiently and effectively, is able to provide the user focus identified in Standards 1 - 16 and is able to meet the requirements of regulation and the standards.

This means that the infrastructure of the business must be sound, operating from premises that are suitable and equipped for the purpose. A business or operational plan is required to ensure that there is strategic planning for the on-going operation and stability of the business. The management structure of the organisation must be appropriate for the effective management of a dispersed workforce, working in stressful and responsible situations, primarily on their own in other peoples own home. The ratio of managers to staff must reflect this and the complexity of the care needs of service users, ie the more complex the level of need the lower the ratio should be of managers to staff All staff must also be employed on a contractual basis with clarity about their areas of responsibility.

Complaints and Quality Assurance

The delivery of effective personal care services to people living in their own home requires a clear infrastructure which identifies each stage of the process of service delivery and provides policies and procedures which support practice.

The delivery of the service and meeting the nationally required standards must be supported by continuous monitoring and evaluation. Each organisation will be required to have a robust mechanism in place for ensuring the quality of the services it is providing and taking the action necessary if the service falls below the standards identified.

Each organisation is also required to have a robust system in place to enable service users and/or their advocates or family carers, to make a formal complaint about the service and for the complaint to be investigated promptly and any necessary action taken. It should be remembered that the majority of people who receive care in their own home are extremely reluctant to complain, even when they have very valid reasons to do so, for fear that the service may be taken away from them. For this reason it is important that the process for making a complaint is accessible, transparent and straighifOrward. The process should include the giving of compliments as well as making complaints so that the whole process is seen and experienced by service users as positive and constructive and not negative and punitive.

(See regulations 20, 21, 22 and 23)

Business premises, management and planning

OUTCOME: Service users receive a consistent, well managed and planned service

STANDARD 22 (See regulation 22)

22.1 **The business operates from permanent premises and there is a management structure in place, including clear lines of accountability, which enables the agency to deliver services effectively on a day to day basis, in accordance with the agency's business plan.**

22.2 The service is managed and provided from sound and permanent premises which are suitable and designated for the purpose, provide a safe working environment for staff and include the provision of private space for confidential meetings.

22.3 The premises are located appropriately for the management and provision of domiciliary care to the people it serves.

22.4 The premises contain equipment and resources necessary for the efficient and effective management of the service.

22.5 The management structure reflects the size of the agency and the volume and complexity of the care provided.

22.6 The registered provider is able to demonstrate there is adequate staff cover for the operation of the agency.

Finanicial procedures

OUTCOME: The continuity of the service provided to service users is safeguarded by the accounting and financial procedures of the agency

STANDARD 23 (See regulations 23 and 26)

23.1 **The registered person ensures that sound accounting and other financial procedures are adopted to ensure the effective and efficient running of the business and its continued financial viability.**

23.2 Systems are in place so that accurate calculation can be made of the charges for the service, to submit invoices regularly and to identify and follow-up any late payment.

23.3 Where audited accounts are not available, annual accounts are completed by a qualified accountant for the purpose of regulation and inspection.

23.4 Insurance cover is sufficient to protect the agency's assets and liabilities. Including the agency's legal liabilities to any and all employees and third party persons to a limit of indemnity commensurate with the level and extent of activities undertaken.

23.5 Assets insurance cover is against any loss or damage, including business interruption costs and for replacement as new of buildings, fixtures, fittings and equipment.

Record Keeping

OUTCOME: The rights and best interests of service users are safeguarded by the agency keeping accurate and up-to-date records

STANDARD 24 (See regulation 19)

24.1 **The agency maintains all the records required for the protection of service users and the efficient running of the business for the requisite length of time including:**

- financial records detailing all transactions of the business

- personal file on each service user *

- personnel files on each member of staff

- interviews of applicants for posts who are subsequently employed

- accident report record (see Standard 11.4) *

- record of incidents of abuse or suspected abuse (including use of restraint) and action taken (see Standards 14 and 18.9)

- record of complaints and compliments and action taken (see Standard 26)

- records of disciplinary and grievance procedures (see Standard 18)

- records kept in the home of service users (see Standard 16) *

(* except for employment agency solely introducing workers)

24.2 All records are secure, up to date and in good order and are constructed, maintained and used in accordance with the Data Protection Act 1998, and other statutory requirements, and are kept for the requisite length of time.

24.3 Consistent and standard personal data are kept on all service users being cared for by the agency (See appendix F), except for employment agencies solely introducing workers.

24.4 Service users or their representatives have access to their records and information about them held by the agency and are facilitated in obtaining access when necessary (see Standard 9).

Policies and procedures

OUTCOME: The service user's rights, health, and best interests are safeguarded by robust policies and procedures which are consistently implemented and constantly monitored by the agency

STANDARD 25

25.1 **The agency implements a clear set of policies and procedures to support practice and meet the requirements of legislation, which are dated, and monitored, as part of the quality assurance process. The policies and procedures are reviewed and amended annually or more &equently if necessary. (See appendix G).**

25.2 Staff understand and have access to up-to-date copies of all policies, procedures and codes of practice, and service users have access to relevant information on the policies and procedures and other documents in appropriate formats.

Complaints and compliments

OUTCOME: Service users and their relatives or representatives are confident that their complaints will be listened to, taken seriously and acted upon

STANDARD 26 (See regulation 20)

26.1 **The registered person ensures that there is an easily understood, well publicised and accessible procedure to enable service users, their relatives or representative to make a complaint or compliment and for complaints to be investigated.**

26.2 The procedure includes the stages and timescales for the process.

26.3 Positive action is taken to encourage, enable and empower service users to use the complaints and compliments procedure including access to appropriate interpretation and methods of communication.

26.4 All complaints are acknowledged in an appropriate form and the investigation commenced within the period specified in the information given to users.

26.5 Service users are kept informed at each and every stage of the investigatory process and are given information on the appeals procedure and for referring a complaint, to the regional office of the National Care Standards Commission, at any stage if they so wish.

26.6 A record is kept of all complaints and compliments including details of the investigation and action taken; this record is also kept on the personal file of the service user kept in the agency and on the home care or support workers personnel record.

26.7 There is a system in place to analyse and identify any pattern of complaints.

Quality Assurance

OUTCOME: The service is run in the best interests of its service users

STANDARD 27 (See regulation 21)

27.1   **There is an effective system for Quality Assurance based on the outcomes for service users, in which standards and indicators to be achieved are clearly defined and monitored on a continuous basis by care and support staff and their line managers.**

27.2   Regulatory standards and other relevant service standards and indicators, eg National Occupational Standards and indicators for the Performance Assessment Framework, are incorporated into the quality assurance (QA) system.

27.3   There is a process and a procedure for consulting with service users and their carers about the care service on a regular basis and assuring quality and monitoring performance including:

- an annual visit to all service users undertaken by a supervisor or manager and combined, where appropriate, with a review of the service user plan (Standard 7) or monitoring the performance of the care or support worker (Standard 21) *

- regular supervision meetings between the line manager and care and support workers (See standard 21) *

- annual survey of service users, their relatives or representative where appropriate to obtain their views and opinions of the service

- checks on records, timesheets etc

* Except for employment agencies solely introducing workers.

27.4   Care and support workers know the standard of service they are required to provide and monitor and meet the standard on a continuous basis.

27.5   The outcome from the QA process is published annually, supplied to the NCSC and made available to users, their family or representatives, and all stakeholders in the agency.

27.6   Standards and the QA process are reviewed and revised as necessary, on an annual basis.

Appendices

A   Glossary of terms

Abuse

Single or repeated act or lack of appropriate action occurring within any relationship where there is an expectation of trust which causes harm or distress to an older person [Action on Elder Abuse] including physical, emotional, verbal, financial, sexual, racial abuse, neglect and abuse through the misapplication of drugs.

Care Assessment

Collection and interpretation of data to determine an individual's need for health, personal and social care and support services, undertaken with the individual, his/her supporter, and relevant professionals.

Care Manager

The person responsible for undertaking the assessment of need, developing and co-ordinating the service user's plan, for monitoring its progress and for staying in regular contact with the service user and everyone involved.

Care Plan

A written statement, regularly updated, and agreed by all parties, setting out the health and social care and support that a service user requires in order to achieve specific outcomes and meet the particular needs of each service user.

Care Programme Approach (CPA)

The formal process of assessing needs for services for people with mental health problems prior to and after discharge from hospital.

Care Worker

A person who works on either a paid or a voluntary basis for an organisation which provides personal domiciliary care services to people who live in their own homes

Contract

Written agreement between the service user and the domiciliary care provider, setting out the terms and conditions, and rights and responsibilities, of both parties, and including the Individual Plan of Care.

Independent advocate

An individual who is independent of any of the statutory agencies involved in purchasing or provision of care in, or the provision or regulation of the domiciliary care service, who acts on behalf of and in the interests of a service user [who feels unable to represent him / herself when dealing with professionals.] Self-advocates are trained and supported to represent their own views.

Intermediate care

A short period (normally no longer than six weeks) of intensive rehabilitation and treatment to enable service users to return home following (or to avoid) hospitalisation, or to prevent admission to long term residential care.

Outcome

The end result of the service provided by a care provider to a service user, which can be used to measure the effectiveness of the service.

Personal care

Includes assistance with bodily functions where required.

Physical intervention

A method of responding to violence or aggressive behaviour which involves a degree of direct physical force to limit or restrict movement or mobility.

Policy

An operational statement of intent which helps staff make sound decisions and take actions which are legal, consistent with the aims of the service, and in the best interests of service users.

Procedure

The steps taken to fulfil a policy.

Registered manager

Senior staff member (who may be the owner) who is responsible for managing the provision of domiciliary care on a daily basis, and is registered with the National Care Standards Commission to do so.

Representative

A person acting on behalf of a service user, who may be a relative or friend.

Service user

Person who is receiving the care service.

Service User Plan

A detailed plan that is developed between the service user and the representative of the agency providing the care which identifies the way in which the care is to be provided and the activities to be undertaken. The Service User Plan arises from the needs assessment, the care plan and the risk and manual handling risk assessment.

Standard

A measure by which quality is judged.

Support worker

A care worker who enables people, generally adults with learning disabilities, physical disabilities, sensory impairment or mental health problems, to maximise their own abilities and independence.

Volunteer

People working without pay, or for expenses only,

B   Content of the code of conduct of the agency

The Code covers:

- compliance with the philosophy of care (privacy, dignity, maintaining independence)

- confidentiality of information

- limits of responsibility

- provision of non-discriminatory practice

- receiving sexual or racial harassment

- health and safety *

- moving and handling

- prevention of any form of abuse

- dealing with accidents & emergencies

- handling and administering medicines

- handling money and financial matters on behalf of a service user *

- acceptance of gifts and legacies

- dress code, *

- use of protective clothing

- protocols and procedures for entering and leaving the home

- personal safety and out of hours working

- not smoking, drinking alcohol or taking illegal substances whilst on duty

- ways in which staff and managers may raise concerns about the management and provision of the service including disclosure of bad practice

- maintaining accurate records

- other relevant policies and procedures

* Except for employment agencies solely introducing workers

C   Content of the induction programme

Induction may be undertaken in a number of different ways:

- a formal course or programme of learning

- shadowing or working alongside an experienced colleague

- completion of a workbook, checklists and other forms of open learning

- a combination of all three

Content should include the following:

- the nature of personal care and the basic skills required

- core values, including providing a 'needs-led' service

- code of personal conduct (see appendix B)

- terms and conditions of employment including disciplinary and grievance procedures

- the requirements of legislation

- policies and working practices of the organisation

- health and safety training including an introduction to manual handling, infection control and fire procedures (see appendix D)

- general health of service users and the role of care and support staff in monitoring their health on an on-going basis.

- communication skills

- prevention of any form of abuse or exploitation of the person receiving care or support and 'whistle-blowing

- anti-discriminatory practice including cultural awareness

- standards to which they should work (including the implications of these standards)

- confidentiality

- gifts and bequests

- principal activities which must not be undertaken

- contextual knowledge about the organisation for which they are working

- quality assurance and monitoring

For managers the induction process should include an introduction to:

- Recruitment and selection

- Supervision and performance appraisal

- Health and safety for managers

- Risk and manual handling risk assessment

- Monitoring practice and quality assurance

D   Content of health and safety training

Health and safety issues are covered in the induction programme including:

* clear statement and parameters of responsibility of care staff and employer

* guidance on appropriate clothing & footwear

* procedure for reporting and recording accidents to service users and care staff

* dealing with violent incidents (or potential incidents) and challenging behaviour

* personal safety and violence prevention towards staff

* dealing with sexual and/or racial harassment

* control of substances hazardous to health

* moving and handling

* first aid (as appropriate to the agency's service users)

* basic hygiene and infection control including dealing with bodily fluids and incontinence management

* food preparation, storage and hygiene

* policy and parameters of responsibility in relation to administering of medication

* notification of transmittable diseases and implications for confidentiality, protection etc

* wearing and use of protective clothing

* risk assessment including common hazards in the home

* maintaining privacy & respect when using equipment, eg hoists

* health and safety implications for people with special needs

* dealing with pets, pests and infestation

* reporting of concerns or faulty equipment

* the rights of users to take risks

* action to take in an emergency situation (as appropriate to the agency's service users)

E   Topics requiring specialist training and advice

Specialist training would normally be expected for working with:

- people from ethnic minority communities and/or religious groups

- children and their families including child protection and prevention/detection of child abuse

- people with special communication needs

- people with sensory loss

- people with dual sensory impairment

- older people with complex health and care needs

- people with a terminal illness

- people who have had a stroke

- people who have learning disabilities

- people with mental health problems including people subject to Guardianship and Supervision Orders under the Mental Health Act

- people with infectious or contagious diseases

- people with dementia

- people with challenging behaviours

F   Data kept on all service users

(not applicable to employment agencies solely introducing workers)

- name, address, date of birth, telephone no.

- preferred form of address

- name, address, telephone no. of next of kin and main carer or person closest to user

- name, address, telephone no. of GP

- name, address, telephone no. of person & organisation providing care

- name, address, telephone no. of care manager or other person responsible for arranging the provision of care (if applicable)

- date of commencement of the service

- date of termination of service - if known

- record of original assessment of need

- date or review/reassessment of service

- outcomes to be achieved for the service user by providing the care.

- detail of the care activities and service to be provided

- detail of the risk assessment including manual handling and any particular requirements arising from it

- any particular or special needs

- medication plan (if appropriate)

- other health care issues if known

- involvement of service user or carer in the provision and direction of their care

The length of time records should be kept include:

- 80 years - Records relating to children

- 40 years - Employment records

- 7 years - Accounts and financial transactions

- 3 years - Interviews of applicants for posts who are subsequently employed

- 6 months for applicants for posts who are not subsequently employed

G   Policies and procedures of the agency

The policies and procedures encompass the following areas:

- statement of purpose and aims and objectives of the organisation

- conditions of engagement including travel expenses, insurance etc

- contract & job description

- range of activities undertaken - and limits of responsibility

- personal safety whilst at work

- standards for quality assurance

- confidentiality of information

- provision of non-discriminatory practice

- equal opportunities, sexual or racial harassment

- health and safety

- moving and handling

- dealing with accidents & emergencies

- disclosure of abuse and bad practice

- data protection and subject access

- assisting with medication

- handling money and financial matters on behalf of a service user

- maintaining the records in the home

- acceptance of gifts and legacies

- dealing with violence & aggression

- entering & leaving a service user's home

- safe keeping of keys

- complaints & compliments

- discipline and grievance

- training and staff development

National minimum standards for...

Domiciliary care agencies

Bibliography and good practice guides

General

- Carefully- A Handbook for Home Care Assistants, 2nd Edition Lesley Bell, Age Concern England 1999 ISBN 086242 285 X

- Managing Carefully - A Guide for Home Care Managers, Lesley Bell, Age Concern England 1996 ISBN 0 86242 185 3

SCA Practice guides

- Code of Practice for Social Care

- The Social Care Task - Improving the Quality of Life

- The UKHCA Code of Practice, United Kingdom Home Care Association

User Focused services

- Culture, Religion and Patient Care in a Multi-ethnic society, A. Henley and J. Schott, Age Concern 1999 ISBN 0862422310

- Caring for Ethnic Minority Elders: a guide, Yasmin Alibhai- Brown, Age Concern 1998 ISBN 0862421888

BADCO Good Practice Guidlines

- Charter of Rights for Home Care Users

- Professional/Personal Boundaries

SCA Practice guide

- Contracts and Agreements in Social Care

UKHCA Document

- Choosing Care in Your Own Home (leaflet)

Personal Care

Pharmacist support for home carers (formerly known as home helps), Pharmacy Community Care Liaison Group, The Pharmaceutical Journal, Volume 260, pp 879-882, June 13 1998.

BADCO Good Practice Guidlines

- Professional/Personal Boundaries

- Medication

- Working in Home Care with Dementia

SCA Practice guides

- Positively Valuing People in Social Care

- Enabling, Participation and Empowerment

- Action Check List for Anti-Racist Practice in Social Care

- Keyworking in Social Care

UKHCA Document

- The Home Care Worker's Handbook

Protection

- No Secrets, Department of Health 2000

- Elder Abuse: Critical issues in policy and practice, Age Concern ISBN 0862422485

Action on elder abuse

- The Home Front, video training package for ZI occupational standard in care
  Code No.1500-283

- Where's the Harm: Elder abuse or not? Video training package
  Code No.1500-282

- **Papers and leaflets**

  - The abuse of older people at home

  - Speaking out on elder abuse

  - Bags of money

  - The great taboo

- Working with Care - Health and Safety in Home Care, Joint Advisory Group of Domiciliary Care Associations 1996

- Working Safely, Suzy Lamplugh Trust

BADCO Good Practice Guildlines

- Personal Safety for Home Care Staff

- Safe Hygiene Practice

- Handling Service User's Finances and Valuables

SCA Practice Guides

- Dealing with Violence in Care Settings

- Recording and Reporting in Social Care

UKHCA Documents

- UKHCA Policy on Administration of Medicines

- Managing Finance: UKH CA Guidelines

- UKHCA Health & Safety Factsheet

- UKHCA Factsheets on MRSA, H IV & Aids, Pressures sores etc.

Managers and Staff

BADCO Good Practice Guildlines

- Code of Practice for the Management of Domiciliary Care

- Professional/Personal Boundaries BADCO Leaflet

- Managing Absence

- Staff Support and Supervision

- Caring for Staff

SCA Practice Guides

- Selecting Staff for Social Care

- Induction Training for Social Care

- Supervision in Social Care

UKHCA Documents

- Training & Matching Care Staff to Perform Specific Tasks - UKHCA Guidelines

Organisation and running of the Business

- Home Care, The Business of Caring, Lesley Bell & Linda How, Age Concern England 1996 ISBN 086242 2124

- A Framework for the Development of Standards for the Provision of Domiciliary Care – Quality Assurance in Domiciliary Care, Joint Advisory Group of Domiciliary Care Associations

SCA Practice Guides

- Recording and Reporting in Social Care

- Complaints in Social Care

- Harassment, Discrimination and Bullying

- Suspending Staff from their Duties

UKHCA Documents

- UKHCA Complaints Procedure and Complaints Procedure for the use of clients.

Action on Elder Abuse Publications are available from

AEA, Astral House, 1268 London Road, London SW16 4ER Tel: 02087647648 Fax: 02086794074 email: aea@ace.org.uk

Age Concern Publications are available from

Age Concern Books, PO Box 232, Newton Abbot, Devon TQ12 4XQ Tel: 08704422044 Fax: 01626364463 email: books@ace.org.uk

BADCO Leaflets are available from

Norcroft Farm, Seighford, Staffs ST18 9PQ. Tel: 01189772878

Jag Booklets are available from

SCA - see address below

Pharmaceutical Journal reference available from

Karen Turnham, Policy Support Unit, Royal Pharmaceutical Society of Great Britain, 1 Lambeth High St, London SE1 7JN
Tel: 02075722218 Fax: 0207793 1923 email: kturnham@rpsgb.org.uk

SCA Publications are available from

Thornton House, Hook Road, Surbiton, Surrey KT6 5AR
Tel: 0208 397 1411 Fax: 0208 397 1436 email: sca@scaed.demon.co.uk

UKHCA Publications are available from

5 Beeches Avenue, Carshalton Beeches, Surrey SM5 3NW
Tel: 0208 288 1551 Fax: 0208 288 1550

STATUTORY INSTRUMENTS

2002 No.3214

SOCIAL CARE, ENGLAND

The Domiciliary Care Agencies Regulations 2002

Made - - - -	*2002*
Laid before Parliament	*2002*
Coming into force - -	*1st April 2003*

ARRANGEMENT OF REGULATIONS
PART I – GENERAL

PART II – REGISTERED PERSONS

PART III – CONDUCT OF DOMICILIARY CARE AGENCIES

Chapter 1
Quality of service provision

Chapter 2
Premises

Chapter 3
Financial matters

Chapter 4
Notices to be given to the Commission

PART IV - MISCELLANEOUS

SCHEDULES

The Secretary of State for Health, in exercise of powers conferred on him by sections 4(6), 22(1), (2)(a) to (d), and (f) to (j), (5)(a) and (7)(a) to (h) and (j), 25,34(1),35 and 118(5) to (7) of the Care Standards Act 2000(a) and of all other powers enabling him in that behalf,

---

(a) 2000 c.14. The powers are exercisable by the appropriate Minister. who is defined in section 121(1). in relation to England. Scotland and Northern Ireland, as the Secretary of State, and in relation to Wales, as the National Assembly for Wales. Prescribed and regulations are defined in section 121(1) of the Act.

having consulted such persons as he considers appropriate(**a**), hereby makes the following Regulations:

PART I

GENERAL

Citation, commencement and application

1. (1) These Regulations may be cited as the Domiciliary Care Agencies Regulations 2002 and shall come into force on 1st April 2003.

(2) These Regulations apply to domiciliary care agencies in England only.

Interpretation

2. (1) In these Regulations

the Act means the Care Standards Act 2000;

agency means a domiciliary care agency;

agency premises means the premises from which the activities of an agency are carried on;

direct service provider means a provider who supplies a domiciliary care worker who is employed by, and who acts for and under the control of, the provider;

domiciliary care worker means a person who

(a) is employed by the agency to act for, and under the control of, another person;

(b) is introduced by an agency to a service user for employment by him; or

(c) is employed by a direct service provider,

in a position which is concerned with the provision of personal care in their own homes for persons who by reason of illness, infirmity or disability are unable to provide it for themselves without assistance;

organisation means a body corporate or any unincorporated association other than a partnership;

registered manager, in relation to an agency, means a person who is registered under Part II of the Act as the manager of the agency;

registered person, in relation to an agency, means any person who is registered as the provider or the manager of the agency;

registered provider, in relation to an agency, means a person who is registered under Part II of the Act as the person carrying on the agency; responsible individual shall be construed in accordance with regulation 7(2);

service user means any person for whom an agency

(a) supplies a domiciliary care worker who is employed by the agency (including domiciliary care workers supplied by a direct service provider); or

(b) provides services for the purpose of supplying him with a domiciliary care worker for employment by him;

service user s guide means the guide produced in accordance with regulation 5(1);

statement of purpose means the written statement compiled in accordance with regulation 4(1).

(**a**) See section 22(9) of the Care Standards Act 2000 for the requirement to consult.

(2) In these Regulations, references to the supply of a domiciliary care worker mean

    (a) the supply of a domiciliary care worker who is employed by an agency to act for and under the control of another person;

    (b) the introduction of a domiciliary care worker by an agency to a service user for employment by him; and

    (c) the supply of a domiciliary care worker employed by a direct service provider to a service user.

(3) In these Regulations, the terms employed and employment include employment under a contract of service or a contract for services, or otherwise than under a contract and whether or not for payment.

Excepted undertakings

3. °For the purposes of the Act, an undertaking is excepted from the definition of domiciliary care agency in section 4(3) of the Act if the undertaking is carried on by an individual who

    (a) carries it on otherwise than in partnership with others;

    (b) is not employed by an organisation to carry it on; and

    (c) does not employ any other person for the purpose of the undertaking.

Statement of purpose

4. (1) °The registered person shall compile in relation to the agency a written statement (in these Regulations referred to as the statement of purpose) which shall consist of a statement as to the matters listed in Schedule 1.

(2) The registered person shall supply a copy of the statement of purpose to the Commission and shall make a copy of it available on request for inspection at the agency premises by every service user and any person acting on behalf of a service user .

(3) Nothing in regulation 22 shall require or authorise the registered person to contravene, or not to comply with

    (a) any other provision of these Regulations; or

    (b) the conditions for the time being in force in relation to the registration of the registered person under Part II of the Act.

Service user s guide

5. (1) The registered person shall produce a service user s guide which shall include

    (a) a summary of the statement of purpose;

    (b) the terms and conditions in respect of the services to be provided to servIce users, including as to the amount and method of payment of fees;

    (c) a summary of the complaints procedure established in accordance with regulation 20; and

    (d) the address and telephone number of the Commission.

(2) The registered person shall make a copy of the service user s guide available on request for inspection at the agency premises by every service user and any person acting on behalf of a servIce user.

Review of statement of purpose and service user s guide

6.   The registered person shall
> (a) keep under review and, where appropriate, revIse the statement of purpose and the service user s guide; and
>
> (b) notify the Commission of any material revision within 28 days.

PART II

REGISTERED PERSONS

Fitness of registered provider

7. (1) A person shall not carry on an agency unless he is fit to do so.

(2) A person is not fit to carry on an agency unless the person
> (a) is an individual, who carries on the agency
>> (i)   otherwise than in partnership with others, and he satisfies the requirements set out in paragraph (3);
>>
>> (ii) in partnership with others, and he and each of his partners satisfies the requirements set out in paragraph (3);
>
> (b) is a partnership, and each of the partners satisfies the requirements set out in paragraph (3);
>
> (c) is an organisation and
>> (i)   the organisation has given notice to the Commission of the name, address and position in the organisation of an individual (in these Regulations referred to as the responsible individual) who is a director, manager, secretary or other officer of the organisation and is responsible for supervising the management of the agency; and
>>
>> (ii) that individual satisfies the requirements set out in paragraph (3).

(3) The requirements are that
> (a) he is of integrity and good character;
>
> (b) he is physically and mentally fit to carry on the agency; and
>
> (c) full and satisfactory information is available in relation to him in respect of each of the matters specified in Schedule 2.

(4) A person shall not carry on an agency if
> (a) he has been adjudged bankrupt or sequestration of his estate has been awarded and (in either case) he has not been discharged and the bankruptcy order has not been annulled or rescinded; or
>
> (b) he has made a composition or arrangement with his creditors and has not been discharged in respect of it.

Appointment of manager

8. (1) The registered provider shall appoint an individual to manage the agency where
> (a) there is no registered manager in respect of the agency; and
>
> (b) the registered provider
>> (i)   is an organisation or a partnership; or
>>
>> (ii) is not a fit person to manage an agency; or
>>
>> (iii) is not, or does not intend to be, in full-time day to day charge of the agency.

(2) Where the registered provider appoints a person to manage the agency, he shall forthwith give notice to the Commission of

    (a) the name of the person so appointed; and

    (b) the date on which the appointment is to take effect.

Fitness of manager

9. (1)° A person shall not manage an agency unless he is fit to do so.

  (2) A person is not fit to manage an agency unless

    (a) he is of integrity and good character;

    (b) having regard to the size of the agency, the statement of purpose and the number and needs of the service users

      (i) he has the qualifications, skills and experience necessary to manage the agency; and

      (ii) he is physically and mentally fit to do so; and

    (c) full and satisfactory information is available in relation to him in respect of each of the matters specified in Schedule 2.

Registered person - general requirements and training

10.(1) The registered provider and the registered manager shall, having regard to the size of the agency, the statement of purpose and the number and needs of the service users, carry on or (as the case may be) manage the agency with sufficient care, competence and skill.

  (2) If the registered provider is

    (a) an individual, he shall undertake;

    (b) an organisation, it shall ensure that the responsible individual undertakes; or

    (c) a partnership, it shall ensure that one of the partners undertakes, from time to time such training as is appropriate to ensure that he has the experience and skills necessary for carrying on the agency.

  (3) The registered manager shall undertake from time to time such training as is appropriate to ensure that he has the experience and skills necessary for managing the agency.

Notification of offences

11.   Where the registered person or the responsible individual is convicted of any criminal offence, whether in England and Wales or elsewhere, he shall forthwith give notice in writing to the Commission of

    (a) the date and place of the conviction;

    (b) the offence of which he was convicted; and

    (c) the penalty imposed on him in respect of the offence.

PART III
CONDUCT OF DOMICILIARY CARE AGENCIES

CHAPTER 1

QUALITY OF SERVICE PROVISION

Fitness of domiciliary care workers supplied by an agency

12. Ihe registered person shall ensure that no domiciliary care worker is supplied by the agency unless

    (a) he is of integrity and good character;

    (b) he has the experience and skills necessary for the work that he is to perform;

    (c) he is physically and mentally fit for the purposes of the work which he is to perform; and

    (d) full and satisfactory information is available in relation to him in respect of each of the matters specified in Schedule 3.

Conduct of agency

13. Where the agency is acting otherwise than as an employment agency(a), the registered person shall make suitable arrangements to ensure that the agency is conducted, and the personal care arranged by the agency, is provided

    (a) so as to ensure the safety of service users;

    (b) so as to safeguard service users against abuse or neglect;

    (c) so as to promote the independence of service users;

    (d) so as to ensure the safety and security of service users property, including their homes;

    (e) in a manner which respects the privacy, dignity and wishes of service users, and the confidentiality of information relating to them; and

    (f) with due regard to the sex, religious persuasion, racial origin, and cultural and linguistic background and any disability of service users, and to the way in which they conduct their lives.

Arrangements for the provision of personal care

14.(1) Paragraphs (2) to (12) apply only to the supply of domiciliary care workers to service users by an agency which is acting otherwise than as an employment agency.

    (2) The registered person shall, after consultation with the service user, prepare a written plan (the service user plan) which shall specify

        (a) the service user s needs in respect of which personal care is to be provided;

        (b) how those needs are to be met by the provision of personal care.

    (3) The registered person shall

        (a) make the service user plan available to the service user;

        (b) keep the service user plan under review;

        (c) where appropriate, and after consultation with the service user, or if consultation with the service user is not practicable, after consultation with a person acting on behalf of the service user, revise the service user plan; and

(d) notify the service user or, where applicable, the person acting on his behalf, of any such revision.

(4) The registered person shall, so far as is practicable, ensure that the personal care which the agency arranges to be provided to any service user meets the service user s needs specified in the service user plan prepared in respect of him.

(5) The registered person shall, for the purpose of providing personal care to service users, so far as is practicable

(a) ascertain and take into account their wishes and feelings;

(b) provide them with comprehensive information and suitable choices as to the personal care that may be provided to them; and

(c) encourage and enable them to make decisions with respect to such personal care.

(6) The registered person shall ensure that where the agency arranges the provision of personal care to a service user, the arrangements shall

(a) specify the procedure to be followed after an allegation of abuse, neglect or other harm has been made;

(b) specify the circumstances in which a domiciliary care worker may administer or assist in the administration of the service user s medication, or any other tasks relating to the service user s health care, and the procedures to be adopted in such circumstances;

(c) include arrangements to assist the service user with mobility in his home, where required; and

(d) specify the procedure to be followed where a domiciliary care worker acts as agent for, or receives money from, a service user.

(7) The registered person shall make arrangements for the recording, handling, safe keeping, safe administration and disposal of medicines used in the course of the provision of personal care to service users.

(8) The registered person shall make suitable arrangements, including training, to ensure that domiciliary care workers operate a sate system of working, including in relation to lifting and . . movIng service users.

(9) The registered person shall make arrangements, by training or by other measures, to prevent service users being harmed or suffering abuse or being placed at risk of harm or abuse.

(10) The registered person shall ensure that no service user is subject to physical restraint unless restraint of the kind employed is the only practicable means of securing the welfare of that or any other service user and there are exceptional circumstances.

(11) On any occasion on which a service user is subject to physical restraint by a person who works as a domiciliary care worker for the purposes of the agency, the registered person shall record the circumstances, including the nature of the restraint.

(a) See section 121(1) of the Care Standards Act 2000 for the definition of employment agency.

(12) The procedure referred to in paragraph (6)(a) shall in particular provide for

    (a) written records to be kept of any allegation of abuse, neglect or other harm and of the action taken in response; and

    (b) the Commission to be notified of any incident reported to the police, not later than 24 hours after the registered person

        (i)   has reported the matter to the police; or

        (ii) is informed that the matter has been reported to the police.

(13) The registered person shall ensure that any personal information about a service user for whom a domiciliary care worker is supplied by the agency is not disclosed to any member of the agency s staff unless it is necessary to do so in order to provide an effective service to the service user.

Staffing

15.(1) "Where an agency is acting otherwise than as an employment agency, the registered person shall, having regard to the size of the agency, the statement of purpose and the number and needs of the service users, ensure that

    (a) there is at all times an appropriate number of suitably skilled and experienced persons employed for the purposes of the agency;

    (b) appropriate information and advice are provided to persons employed for the purposes of the agency, and are made available to them at their request, in respect of

        (i)   service users and their needs in respect of personal care; and

        (ii) the provision of personal care to service users;

    (c) suitable assistance and where necessary , appropriate equipment, is provided to persons working for the purposes of the agency, and is made available to them at their request, in respect of the provision of personal care to service users;

    (d) suitably qualified and competent persons are available to be consulted during any period of the day in which a person is working for the purposes of the agency; and

    (e) neither of the following circumstances, that is

        (i)   the employment of any persons on a temporary basis for the purposes of the agency; and

        (ii) any arrangements made for persons to work as domiciliary care workers on a temporary basis for those purposes,

will prevent service users from receiving such continuity of care as is reasonable to meet their needs for personal care.

(2) The registered person shall ensure that each employee of the agency

    (a) receives training and appraisal which are appropriate to the work he is to perform;

    (b) receives suitable assistance, including time off, for the purpose of obtaining qualifications appropriate to such work;

    (c) is provided with a job description outlining his responsibilities.

(3) The registered person shall take such steps as may be necessary to address any aspect of the performance of a domiciliary care worker which is found to be unsatisfactory.

(4) The registered person shall ensure that each employee receives appropriate supervision.

Staff handbook

16.(1) Where the agency is acting otherwise than as an employment agency, the registered person shall prepare a staff handbook and provide a copy to every member of staff.

(2) The handbook prepared in accordance with paragraph (1) shall include a statement as to
- (a) the conduct expected of members of staff, and disciplinary action which may be taken against them;
- (b) the role and responsibilities of domiciliary care workers and other staff;
- (c) record keeping requirements;
- (d) recruitment procedures; and
- (e) training and development requirements and opportunities.

Provision of information to service users

17.(1) The registered person shall ensure that before a domiciliary care worker is supplied to a service user, the service user is informed of
- (a) the name of the domiciliary care worker to be supplied, and the means of contacting him;
- (b) the name of the member of staff of the agency who is responsible for the supply of that domiciliary care worker; and
- (c) where the agency is acting otherwise than as an employment agency, details of how he may contact the registered person, or a person nominated to act on behalf of the registered person.

(2) The registered person shall ensure that the information specified in paragraph (1) is, where appropriate, provided to the service user s relatives or carers.

Identification of workers

18. °Where the agency is acting otherwise than as an employment agency, the registered person shall ensure that every domiciliary care worker supplied by the agency is instructed that, while attending on a service user for the purposes of the provision of personal care, he must present the service user with identification showing his name, the name of the agency and a recent photograph.

Records

19.(1) The registered person shall ensure that the records specified in Schedule 4 are maintained and that they are
- (a) kept up to date, in good order and in a secure manner; and
- (b) retained for a period of not less than three years beginning on the date of the last entry.

(2) The registered person shall ensure that, in addition to the records referred to in paragraph (1), a copy of the service user plan and a detailed record of the personal care provided to the service user are kept at the service user s home and that they are kept up to date, in good order and III a secure manner.

Complaints

20.(1) The registered person shall establish a procedure (the complaints procedure) for considering complaints made to the registered person by a service user or a person acting on behalf of a service user.

(2) The registered person shall supply a written copy of the complaints procedure to every service user and, upon request, to any person acting on behalf of a service user.

(3) The written copy of the complaints procedure shall include

(a) the address and telephone number of the Commission; and

(b) the procedure (if any) which has been notified by the Commission to the registered person for making complaints to the Commission relating to the agency.

(4) The registered person shall ensure that every complaint made under the complaints procedure is fully investigated.

(5) The registered person shall, within the period of 28 days beginning on the date on which the complaint is made, or such shorter period as may be reasonable in the circumstances, inform the person who made the complaint of the action (if any) that is to be taken in response.

(6) The registered person shall maintain a record of each complaint, including details of the investigations made, the outcome and any action taken in consequence and the requirements of regulation 19(1) shall apply to that record.

(7) The registered person shall supply to the Commission at its request a statement containing a summary of the complaints made during the twelve months ending on the date of the request and the action taken in response.

Review of quality of service provision

21.(1) The registered person shall introduce and maintain a system for reviewing at appropriate intervals the quality of personal care which the agency arranges to be provided.

(2) The registered person shall supply to the Commission a report in respect of any review conducted by him for the purposes of paragraph (1) and shall make a copy of the report available on request for inspection at the agency premises by service users and persons acting on behalf of service users.

(3) The system referred to in paragraph (1) shall provide for consultation with service users and persons acting on behalf of service users.

CHAPTER 2
PREMISES

Fitness of premises

22. Subject to regulation 4(3), the registered person shall not use the premises for the purpose of an agency unless the premises are suitable for the purpose of achieving the aims and objectives of the agency set out in the statement of purpose.

CHAPTER 3

FINANCIAL MATTERS

Financial position

23.(1) The registered provider shall carry on the agency in such manner as is likely to ensure that the agency will be financially viable for the purpose of achieving the aims and objectives of the agency set out in the statement of purpose.

(2) The registered person shall, if the Commission so requests, provide the Commission with such information and documents as it may require in order to consider the financial viability of the agency, including

    (a) the annual accounts of the agency, certified by an accountant; and

    (b) a certificate of insurance for the registered provider in respect of liability which may be incurred by him in relation to the agency in respect of death, injury, public liability, damage or other loss.

CHAPTER 4

NOTICES TO BE GIVEN TO THE COMMISSION

Notice of absence

24.(1) Where

    (a) the registered provider, being an individual in full-time day to day charge of the agency; or

    (b) the registered manager,

proposes to be absent from the agency for a continuous period of 28 days or more, the registered person shall give notice in writing to the Commission of the proposed absence.

(2) Except in the case of an emergency, the notice referred to in paragraph (1) shall be given no later than one month before the proposed absence commences, or within such shorter period as may be agreed with the Commission and the notice shall specify

    (a) the length or expected length of the absence;

    (b) the reason for the absence;

    (c) the arrangements which have been made for running the agency during that absence;

    (d) the name, address and qualifications of the person who will be responsible for the agency during that absence; and

    (e) in the case of the absence of the registered manager, the arrangements that have been, or are proposed to be, made for appointing another person to manage the agency during that absence, including the proposed date by which the appointment is to be made.

(3) Where the absence arises as a result of an emergency, the registered person shall give notice of the absence within one week of its occurrence specifying the matters set out in paragraph (2)(a) to (e).

(4) Where

    (a) the registered provider, being an individual in full-time day to day charge of the agency; or

    (b) the registered manager,

has been absent from the agency for a continuous period of 28 days or more, and the Commission has not been given notice of the absence, the registered person shall, without delay, give notice in writing to the Commission of the absence, specifying the matters set out in paragraph (2)(a) to (e).

(5) The registered person shall notify the Commission of the return to duty of the registered provider or (as the case may be) the registered manager not later than 7 days after the date of his return.

Notice of changes

25. The registered person shall give notice in writing to the Commission as soon as it is practicable to do so if any of the following events takes place or are proposed to take place

    (a) a person other than the registered person carries on or manages the agency;

    (b) a person ceases to carry on or manage the agency;

    (c) where the registered person is an individual, he changes his name;

    (d) where the registered provider is a partnership, there is any change in the membership of that partnership;

    (e) where the registered provider is an organisation

        (i) the name or address of the organisation is changed;

        (ii) there is any change of director, manager, secretary or other similar officer of the organisation; and

        (iii) there is any change in the identity of the responsible individual;

    (f) where the registered provider is an individual, a trustee in bankruptcy is appointed;

    (g) where the registered provider is a company or partnership, a receiver, manager , liquidator or provisional liquidator is appointed; or

    (h) the registered provider acquires additional premises for the purposes of the agency.

Appointment of liquidators etc.

26.(1) Any person to whom paragraph (2) applies must

    (a) forthwith notify the Commission of his appointment indicating the reasons for it;

    (b) appoint a manager to take full-time day to day charge of the agency in any case where there is no registered manager; and

    (c) not more than 28 days after his appointment, notify the Commission of his intentions regarding the future operation of the agency.

(2) This paragraph applies to any person appointed as

    (a) the receiver or manager of the property of a company or partnership which is a registered provider in respect of an agency;

    (b) the liquidator or provisional liquidator of a company which is the registered provider in respect of an agency;

    (c) the trustee in bankruptcy of a registered provider in respect of an agency.

Death of registered person

27.(1) If more than one person is registered in respect of an agency, and a registered person dies, the surviving registered person shall without delay notify the Commission of the death in writing.

(2) If only one person is registered in respect of an agency, and he dies, his personal representatives must notify the Commission in writing

    (a) without delay of the death; and

    (b) within 28 days of their intentions regarding the future running of the agency.

(3) The personal representatives of the deceased registered provider may carry on the agency without being registered in respect of it

    (a) for a period not exceeding 28 days; and

    (b) for any further period as may be determined in accordance with paragraph (4).

(4) The Commission may extend the period specified in paragraph (3)(a) by such further period, not exceeding one year, as the Commission shall determine, and shall notify any such determination to the personal representatives in writing.

(5) The personal representatives shall appoint a person to take full-time day to day charge of the agency during any period in which, in accordance with paragraph (3), they carry on the agency without being registered in respect of it.

PART IV
MISCELLANEOUS

Compliance with regulations

28. Where there is more than one registered person in respect of an agency, anything which is required under these Regulations to be done by the registered person shall, if done by one of the registered persons, not be required to be done by any of the other registered persons.

Offences

29.(1) A contravention or failure to comply with regulations 4 to 6 and 11 to 25 shall be an offence.

(2) The Commission shall not bring proceedings against a person in respect of any contravention or failure to comply with those regulations unless

    (a) subject to paragraph (4), he is a registered person;

    (b) notice has been given to him in accordance with paragraph (3);

    (c) the period specified in the notice, within which the registered person may make representations to the Commission, has expired; and

    (d) in a case where, in accordance with paragraph (3)(b), the notice specifies any action that is to be taken within a specified period, the period has expired and the action has not been taken within that period.

(3) Where the Commission considers that the registered person has contravened or failed to comply with any of the provisions of the regulations mentioned in paragraph (1), it may serve a notice on the registered person specifying

    (a) in what respect in its opinion the registered person has contravened any of the regulations, or has failed or is failing to comply with the requirements of any of those regulations;

    (b) where it is practicable for the registered person to take action for the purpose of complying with any of those regulations, the action which, in the opinion of the Commission, the registered person should take for that purpose;

    (c) the period, not exceeding three months, within which the registered person should take any action specified in accordance with sub-paragraph (b);

(d) the period, not exceeding one month, within which the registered person may make representations to the Commission about the notice.

(4) The Commission may bring proceedings against a person who was once, but no longer is, a registered person, in respect of a failure to comply with regulation 19, and for this purpose, references in paragraphs (2) and (3) to a registered person shall be taken to include such a person.

Signed by authority of the Secretary of State for Health

Minister of State,
Department of Health

Date   2002

Regulation 4(1)

SCHEDULE 1
INFORMATION TO BE INCLUDED IN THE STATEMENT OF PURPOSE

1.   The aims and objectives of the agency.

2.   The nature of the services which the agency provides.

3.   The name and address of the registered provider and of any registered manager .

4.   The relevant qualifications and experience of the registered provider and any registered manager .

5.   The range of qualifications of the domiciliary care workers supplied by the agency.

6.   The complaints procedure established in accordance with regulation 20.

Regulations 7(3) and 9(2)

SCHEDULE 2

INFORMATION REQUIRED IN RESPECT OF REGISTERED PROVIDERS AND MANAGERS OF AN AGENCY

1.   Proof of identity, including a recent photograph.

2.   Either

   (a) where the certificate is required for a purpose relating to section 115(5)(ea) of the Police Act 1997 (registration under Part II of the Care Standards Act 2000)(a), or the position falls within section 115(3) or (4) of that Act(b), an enhanced criminal record certificate issued under section 115 of that Act; or

   (b) in any other case, a criminal record certificate issued under section 113 of that Act, including, where applicable, the matters specified in section 113(3A) and 115(6A) of that Act and the following provisions once they are in force, namely section 113(3C)(a) and (b) and section 115(6B)(a) and (b) of that Act(c).

3.   Two written references, including a reference relating to the last period of employment of not less than three months duration.

4.   Where a person has previously worked in a position which involved work with children or vulnerable adults, verification, so far as reasonably practicable, of the reason why he ceased to work in that position.

5.   Documentary evidence of any relevant qualifications and training.

6.   A full employment history , together with a satisfactory written explanation of any gaps in employment.

7.   Details of health record.

8.   Details of registration with or membership of any professional body.

9.   Details of any professional indemnity insurance.

(**a**) Section 115(5)(ea) is inserted by the Care Standards Act 2000, section 104.

(**b**) A position is within section 115(3) if it involves regularly caring for, training, supervising or being in sole charge of persons aged under 18. A position is within section 115(4) if it is of a kind specified in regulations and involves regularly caring for . training, supervising or being in sole charge of persons aged 18 or over.

(**c**) Sections 113(3A) and 115(6A) are added to the Police Act 1997 by section 8 of the Protection of Children Act 1999 (c.14), and amended by sections 104 and 116 of, and paragraph 25 of Schedule 4 to, the Care Standards Act 2000 Sections 113(3C) and 115(68) are added to the Police Act 1997 by section 90 of the Care Standards Act 2000 on a date to be appointed.

Regulation 12

SCHEDULE 3
INFORMATION REQUIRED IN RESPECT OF DOMICILIARY CARE WORKERS

1. Name, address, date of birth and telephone number.

2. Name, address and telephone number of next of kin.

3. Proof of identity, including a recent photograph.

4. Details of any criminal offences

    (a) of which the person has been convicted, including details of any convictions which are spent within the meaning of section 1 of the Rehabilitation of Offenders Act 1974(a) and which may be disclosed by virtue of the Rehabilitation of Offenders (Exceptions) Order 1975(b); or

    (b) in respect of which he has been cautioned by a constable and which, at the time the caution was given, he admitted.

5. Two written references, including a reference relating to the last period of employment of not less than three months duration which involved work with children or vulnerable adults.

6. Where the person has previously worked in a position which involved work with children or vulnerable adults, verification, so far as reasonably practicable, of the reason why he ceased to work in that position.

7. Evidence of a satisfactory knowledge of the English language, where the person s qualifications were obtained outside the United Kingdom.

8. Documentary evidence of any relevant qualifications and training.

9. A full employment history , together with a satisfactory written explanation of any gaps in employment and details of any current employment other than for the purposes of the agency.

10. A statement by the person as to the state ofhis physical and mental health.

11. A statement by the registered provider, or the registered manager, as the case may be, that the person is physically and mentally fit for the purposes of the work which he is to perform.

12. Details of any professional indemnity insurance.

Regulation 19(1)

SCHEDULE 4
RECORDS TO BE MAINTAINED FOR INSPECTION

1. All information provided to the Commission for the purposes of registration in relation to the agency.

(**a**) 1974 c.53.
(**b**) S.I. 1975/1023. Relevant amendments have been made by S.I. 1986/1249, 1986/2268,2001/1192 and 2002/441.

2.   Details of every allegation of abuse, neglect or other harm made against an employee of, or any domiciliary care worker who works for, the agency, including details of the investigations made, the outcome and any action taken in consequence.

3.   Details of any physical restraint used on a service user by a person who works as a domiciliary care worker for the purposes of the agency.

4.   The service user plan devised for each service user in accordance with regulation 14, and a detailed record of the personal care provided to that service user.

EXPLANATORY NOTE
(This note is not part of the Regulations)

These Regulations are made under the Care Standards Act 2000 (the Act), and apply in relation to domiciliary care agencies in England only. Part I of the Act establishes, in relation to England, the National Care Standards Commission (the Commission) and Part II provides for the registration and inspection of establishments and agencies, including domiciliary care agencies, by the Commission. It also provides powers to make regulations governing the conduct of establishments and agencies.

Regulation 3 excepts certain agencies from being a domiciliary care agency.

By regulation 4, each agency must prepare a statement of purpose in relation to the matters set out in Schedule 1 and a service user s guide to the agency (regulation 5). The agency must be carried on in a manner which is consistent with the statement of purpose.

Regulations 7 to 11 make provision about the fitness of the persons carrying on and managing an agency and require satisfactory information to be obtained in relation to the matters specified in Schedule 2. Where the provider is an organisation, it must nominate a responsible individual in respect of whom this information must be available (regulation 7). Regulation 8 prescribes the circumstances where a manager must be appointed in respect of the agency, and regulation 9 makes provision concerning the fitness of the manager. Regulation 10 imposes general requirements in relation to the proper conduct of the agency, and the need for appropriate training.

Part III makes provision in relation to the conduct of agencies, in particular about the quality of services to be provided by an agency. Regulation 12 makes provision about the fitness of domiciliary care workers and requires satisfactory information to be obtained in relation to the matters specified in Schedule 3. Regulations 13 and 14 set out the arrangements that must be made by a registered person relating to the conduct of an agency generally and also the procedures which must be implemented in circumstances where domiciliary care workers are supplied to patients by an agency acting otherwise than as an employment agency. In addition, provision is made as to staffing (regulation 15), the staff handbook (regulation 16), the provision of information to service users (regulation 17), the identification of domiciliary care workers (regulation 18), record keeping (regulation 19 and Schedule 4) and complaints (regulation 20). Provision is also made about the suitability of premises (regulation 22) and the financial management of the agency (regulation 23). Regulations 24 to 27 deal with the giving of notices to the Commission.

Part IV deals with miscellaneous matters. In particular, regulation 29 provides for offences. A breach of regulations 4 to 6 and 11 to 25 may found an offence on the part of the registered person. However, no prosecution may be brought unless the Commission has given notice which sets out in what respect it is alleged he is not complying with a regulation, and what action (if any), and by when, the Commission considers is necessary in order to comply with the regulation.